"Dr. Susanne Bennett has done it again...this time she does a deep dive into the magic of kimchi and its myriad health benefits! Her new book, *The Kimchi Diet*, provides a step by step plan that includes mouthwatering recipes with detailed instructional photos. She makes it easy for you to revive your gut, get rid of chronic symptoms and start feeling great again. This diet is for everyone, and please include your children: it gives them a wonderful head start."

Hyla Cass, MD, Integrative Psychiatrist, author of *8 Weeks to Vibrant Health*

"*The Kimchi Diet* is a game changer! Susanne breaks down a simple and easy to follow program that can completely naturally transform your health and your life. If you're looking for a wonderful way to feed your mind, body, and soul—with zero guesswork—grab a copy of this book today!"

Cynthia Garcia, CEO and Founder of Institute of Transformational Nutrition

"As our science is informing us, our guts are the foundation to our physical, emotional and mental health. We now know that we make more than 80% of our immune cells in our gut and more than 90% of our serotonin. So without our gut being healthy and strong, we can not protect ourselves from many of the chronic diseases such as autoimmune conditions, depression/anxiety, cancer and heart disease. This is why I couldn't be more excited about Dr. Susanne Bennett's new book! She takes improving our gut health to a level that we simply haven't seen before. Her recipes and tools are a game changer! I encourage all of my patients and readers to order her book, *The Kimchi Diet*. I have seen the powerful impact her wisdom and medicine has within days!"

Dawn A. DeSylvia, MD, Founder of The Center for Whole Health

"Dr. Susanne's *The Kimchi Diet* is a powerful guide to ensure that this superfood is an integral part of your daily life. *The Kimchi Diet* gives you the empowerment to use this powerhouse Korean staple—rich with probiotics, antioxidants and immune boosting goodness—as a practical tool to incorporate into your daily practice, so you can take control of your gut, health and future. *The Kimchi Diet* is a simple, delicious and informative book that's a must-have in every kitchen."

Kerry Smith, Certified High-Performance Coach and Founder of The Awakening Trainings

"As a holistic pediatrician and pediatric integrative medicine expert, I know firsthand the power of fermented foods and healing the gut to prevent and reverse chronic illness in our kids and help them thrive—body, mind, & spirit. *The Kimchi Diet* introduces us to this incredible Korean superfood that has the power to kill the flu, lower chronic inflammation, promote healthy weight, improve mood and reduce anxiety. With Dr. Susanne Bennett's groundbreaking book, you'll learn how to make kimchi and incorporate it into your daily and delicious part of your whole family's diet! One of Korea's best-kept health secrets is out, thanks to Dr. Bennett and *The Kimchi Diet!*"

Elisa Song, MD, Holistic pediatrician and Founder of Healthy Kids Happy Kids

"*The Kimchi Diet* is rooted in ancient wisdom and modern science. Dr. Bennett brings to life a traditional superfood that not only nourishes but also transforms health and metabolism."

Dr. Nalini Chilkov, LAc, OMD, Founder of the American Institute of Integrative Oncology Research and Education

"I love *The Kimchi Diet* as it can supercharge any food pattern. Rather than another fad diet, *The Kimchi Diet* combines the wisdom of ancient natural healing with the modern science of the central role of gut health. This book is a great addition to my patient's wellness journeys."

Joel Kahn, MD, FACC, Author of *The Plant Based Solution*

It brings me great pleasure to endorse *The Kimchi Diet*. My father, Emanuel Eliaz, who was a civil engineer and developed in Korea the technology for growing rice on the mountainside, offered me the rare opportunity to live in Seoul in 1974 and 1975. Living on the third floor in Namsan Building B, two stories under us was one of the best Korean restaurants in Seoul. The smell and taste of the kimchi became something we savored and learned to appreciate. In this book, Dr. Bennett brings her passion and commitment to a healthy lifestyle and healing for life by introducing us to the value of fermented foods. With the critical importance of the microbiome, of our interdependent relationship with the microbial universe inside our body and gut unfolding, this book can serve as an important tool to enhance our wellbeing and healing.

Isaac Eliaz, MD, Medical Director of Amitaba Medical Clinic

"Kimchi—which, before now, was a little-understood Korean side dish— is the centerpiece of this wonderful program for health and vitality! Bravo, Dr. Bennett!"

"Dr. Susanne Bennett has done it again! Susanne (Dr. Bennett) consistently brings us the latest and greatest information out there. Her easy to read, casual writing style makes it hard not to read, understand and follow. Gut health is everything, and I always wanted to know much more about fermented foods. Now I have the inside scoop!"

"Our diets have become grossly lacking in diversity in modern life. Meanwhile, we are exposed to antibiotics and herbicides in our food. This has resulted in an epidemic of digestive degradation, and a corresponding increase in obesity and inflammatory disease. Dr. Bennett's brilliant book, *The Kimchi Diet* gets you back in the kitchen, making a traditional food that can restore gut health with little expense or time!"

Dr. Susanne Bennett is one of the most incredible physicians I know. She is thorough, knowledgeable and an amazing healer who practices what she preaches. I am super excited about her new book *The Kimchi Diet*—a labor of love where she shares her wisdom about this wonderful ancient superfood—kimchi. We all know that eating probiotic foods is one of the best ways to heal our digestion and kimchi is one of my favorite probiotic foods! Get ready for some amazing healing. I can't wait to make my own kimchi!

"A wonderful examination of one of the world's most amazing superfoods!"

Dr. Susanne Bennett latest book, *The Kimchi Diet*, will change your life. Once you taste the power of kimchi, your whole body will wake up to it's yummy flavors that satisfies your soul and body. Because of this, you no longer have the need to overeat or walk around the kitchen, opening the refrigerator looking for more food and/or crave junk food like you may have used to. You'll find yourself making healthier food choices effortlessly and as a result, become healthier and leaner. Kimchi is also loaded with beneficial bacteria which helps support a healthy immune system for the entire family. And I love the simple recipes that Dr. Susanne has put together to guide you in making your own kimchi, how cool is that! If you want to do one simple thing to improve your life today, get Dr. Susanne Bennett's book, *The Kimchi Diet* because I can't think of a better person to bring the joyful taste, healthy recipes, knowledge and its tradition of kimchi into your life.

Grace Suh, LAc, Holistic Acupuncturist and someone who can't live without kimchi!

"Dr. Susanne Bennett does a great job explaining the health promoting properties of this mysterious sounding food, kimchi. She teaches us about its history and walks us step by step through the process of how to make a variety of different types of kimchi in her new book, *The Kimchi Diet*. Yes, kimchi doesn't have to contain hot red peppers and be super spicy. Kimchi is a perfect example of the "food as medicine" concept and I can't wait to make my first batch of kimchi! As a Functional Medicine practitioner who specializes in digestive disorders, kimchi can be a perfect addition to help my patients improve their gut bacteria balance, which is crucial for their health."

Dr. Ben Weitz, Sports Chiropractic Physician and Functional Medicine practitioner and host of the Rational Wellness Podcast

"In a world of deprivation diets that repeatedly fail, Dr. Susanne Bennett's *The Kimchi Diet* delivers simple, tasty, daily, dietary additions that ensure our success. By revving up our digestion, decreasing inflammation, helping us lose weight and restoring our emotional balance, *The Kimchi Diet* helps us create more easily, the brilliant health that we all deserve. Dr. Susanne's book showcases the clinical validity of this Korean staple by detailing centuries of cultural proof as well as solid modern science. The Universal Superfood called Kimchi now takes center stage as an essential ingredient in successful weight loss and healing."

Kyrin Dunston, MD, FACOG, Author of *Cracking the Bikini Code: 6 Secrets to Permanent Weight Loss Success* and host of Her Brilliant Health Radio Podcast

THE
KIMCHI
DIET

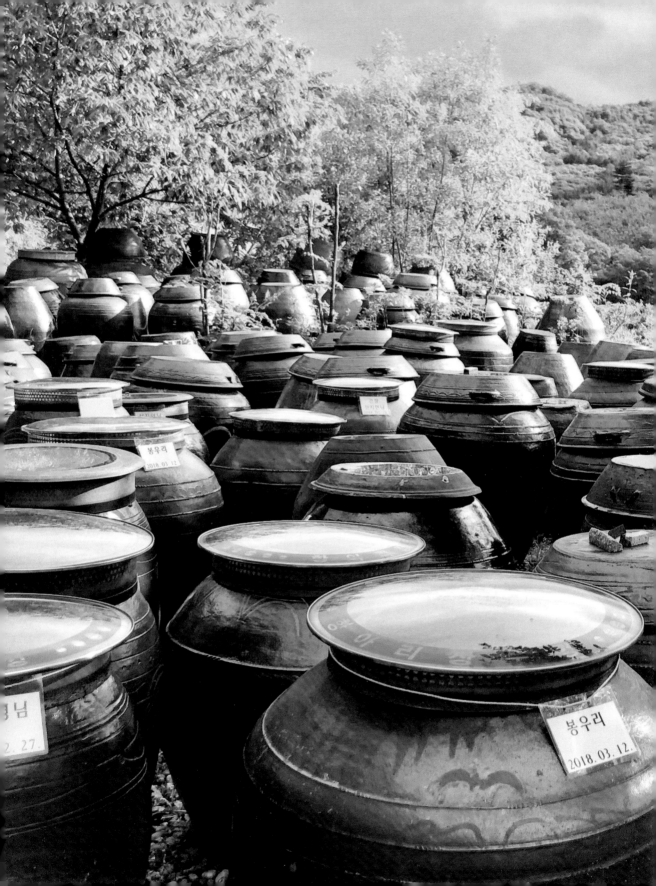

The Kimchi Diet

Revive Your Gut • Get Lean • Live Longer

Dr. Susanne Bennett

The material in this book is for informational purposes only and is a result of years of clinical practice experience by the author. This information is not intended as a substitute for the advice and care by your healthcare professional and do not use this information for diagnosing or treating a health problem or disease. All matters regarding your health require medical supervision.

Neither the author or publisher shall be liable or responsible for any adverse effects allegedly arising from the use of any information or suggestions contained in this book.

Internet addresses and telephone numbers given in this book were accurate at the time it went to press.

Mention of specific products or companies does not imply endorsement by the author or publisher, nor does the mention of these products imply that the companies endorse the book, its author or the publisher.

First Edition: April 2019

ISBN 978-0-997-37351-6
eISBN 978-0-997-37350-9

Published in the United States of America

Photographs by Kelli MacTaggart of MacTaggart Media and Dr. Susanne Bennett
Book Cover Stylized by Cory Gomberg
Book Design by Cosmin Augustin Silaghi and Petre Nicolescu

Printed in China

Wellness for Life Press
1526 14th Street, Suite 111
Santa Monica, CA 90404

thekimchidiet.com
drsusanne.com

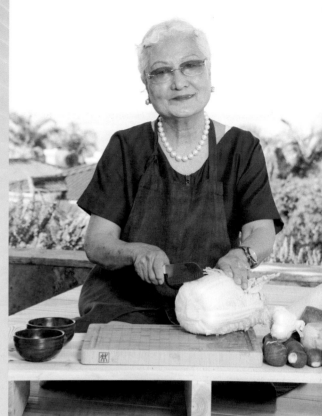
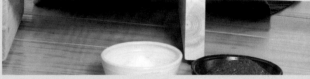

Dedication

This book is dedicated to my 88-years young mother, Suh Jung Hee. The inspiration to write this book started as a project of love—love for my country and heritage, love for my son Cody, love for my family and future generations, and above all, love for my mother, who taught me everything I know about life and the love of kimchi.

Contents

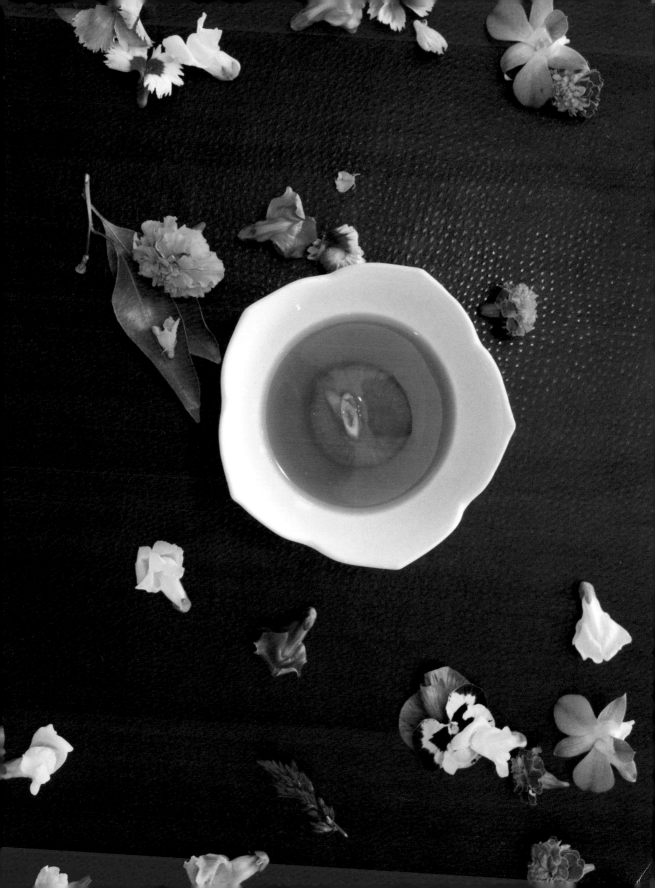

Foreword

by *Dr. Tom O'Bryan*

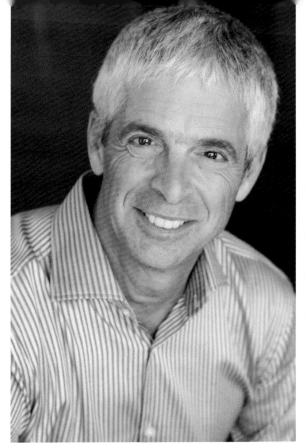

We're going to talk about what scientists now agree is the primary topic in being healthy and preventing disease. No exaggeration—it's primary. Most important. The Big Kahuna. When you understand this topic and what to do about it, you and your family are so much further down the road to a healthy and vibrant disease-reduced life. I don't know of any other topic that has such a magnitude of impact as this one. Because of that, I was honored when my friend Dr. Susanne Bennett asked if I would write the Foreword to her new book, *The Kimchi Diet*.

Whether you speak with the professor of brain neurosurgery at the local university or the massage therapist at the hair salon in the mall down the street, every healthcare practitioner—every single one—knows that in the last 15 to 20 years, an entire new world has been recognized, labeled and studied. With hundreds, no, thousands of research teams around the world working day and night trying to understand this recently-identified-for-the-first-time system of the body, the microbiome has been called *'The Undiscovered Organ'*[1].

Here are a few bullet points about the microbiome:

- The microbiome produces hormones that tell the brain what to do. The term is *'modulates'*, which is a good Scrabble word meaning 'has its hands on the steering wheel, controlling the direction you're going in'. For example, for every message from the brain telling the gut what to do, there are 9 messages from the gut telling the brain what to do. Thus, it's the microbiome that determines how many brain hormones, called neurotransmitters, that you make. And it's your neurotransmitter levels that fuel your different feelings (joy, sadness, happiness, fear...). So in terms of our emotions and feelings, a very rational question is *"who is controlling who?"*

- For every human cell in the body, there are 10 non-human cells in the microbiome. That's correct—the ratio is 10:1. Add up all the bone cells, nerve cells, muscle cells, skin cells...all of the human cells in the body, and there are 10 times more foreign cells in the microbiome coming from archaea, bacteria, viruses and protozoa. So in terms of our body composition, a very rational question is *"who is dominant here?"*

- Scientists have known for decades that our function—every function in our body as far as I know—is controlled by what genes get turned on and what genes are turned off, thereby producing the instructional messengers, the proteins that determine all bodily functions. So a rational question is what turns the genes on and off?

- April 14th, 2003 is recognized as the anniversary date of when the Human Genome was fully identified. The mapping of all of the genes in the human body, which the US government began in 1984, was a tremendous effort that we all thought would unlock the keys to health. Well it didn't. We've learned that we were mistaken about that. Genes do not control the direction of your health. What *happens* to the genes determines the direction of your health. Genes get turned on and genes get turned off. THAT's the key that unlocks the direction of your health. So what turns our genes on and what turns our genes off? What turns on the breast cancer gene? Or the Alzheimer's gene? The answer is the environment around the genes. It's called the epigenome (another good Scrabble word that means 'around the genes').

- There are about 23,000 genes in the Human Genome. We know that in terms of the epigenome, there are 100 to 150 times more genes in the microbiome from the archaea, bacteria, viruses and protozoa than in the human genome. Thus, there's about 2,500,000 to 3,000,000 genes in the epigenome.

- And these bacteria sound like something out of a Star Wars movie or a Klingon community. With names like Akkermansia, Allobaculum, Eubacterium, Clostridium, Klebsiella...you don't know whether to feed them or shoot them! Are they saying *"we come in peace"*, or have they come to conquer? In the last 20 years, doctors had to learn about an entire galaxy inside the body that technology was not sophisticated enough to identify beforehand. We never knew it was there. For example, we were taught that the womb was sterile during pregnancy. Now we know that's the furthest thing from the truth and that the entire maternal (mom, mom's parents and mom's grandparents) line of health strengths and disease vulnerabilities are passed on to the developing baby from mom's microbiome during gestation and birthing.

- You grab a light switch and you have to pull it up or down to turn the light on or off. These microbial genes create the pull on the switch of your human genes, turning them on or off. Actually, it's more of a dimmer switch than an on/off switch. That's why you can slowly reverse diseases (dim down the Alzheimer's gene or the autism genes, etc.). So, who is more dominant here? Who is making more noise?

- And we know that the microbial epigenome surrounds the human genes, infiltrating the inner command centers of the human genome, turning the dimmer up or down. So who is creating the message, working the dimmer switches here in the command center of your human genes? It's all of the construction crew building the movie set, the switchboard operators, the secretaries, the lighting people, the sound people, the camera operators, the runners, the maintenance people (the Akkermansia, the Allobaculum, the Lactobacillus, the Eubacterium, the Bifidobacterium, the Clostridium, the Klebsiella, and the thousand more species that make up the diversity of your microbiome). They're the ones who determine which human genes get turned on and which human genes get turned off. They create the picture—the movie that is playing in your cells.

- Wondering how to prevent activating the Alzheimer's gene? You have to turn the dimmer switch down on the Alzheimer's gene. To do that, you must balance the microbiome. Wondering how to prevent activating the cancer gene that runs in your family? You have to turn the dimmer switch down on the cancer gene. To do that, you must balance the microbiome.

- In your digestive tract, in the tube that goes from the mouth to the other end, this is where most of the bugs—the bacteria and viruses—live. They're the ones that modulate your genetic expression by turning the dimmer switches up or down. Remember the term modulate 'has its hands on the steering wheel, controlling where you're going'? ARE YOU GOING TOWARDS BREAST CANCER, TOWARDS ALZHEIMER'S, TOWARDS...? Or going away from it? Is your dimmer switch for any and every gene turning it brighter? Or dimming it down? Some you want bright. Some you want dim.

- So wait a minute here. Let me get this straight. Are you saying that there is 10 times more cells of archaea, bacteria, viruses and protozoa than human cells. And these cells have 100 to 150 times more genes than the human genome? And these microbiome genes are in the epigenetics (around the human genes)? And it's the epigenetic activity that determines which human genes get turned on and which human genes get turned off? That's a fact, Jack! Please excuse me, I have to have a little bit of fun when doing a deep dive like this.

There are thousands of published articles on the impact of the microbiome on our health. Thousands. Do you get my point? It's the microbiome that has its hands on the steering wheel of how your body functions. What part of your body? Every part of your body. The titles of these few research articles may give you an appreciation of the scope of impact here. And this is just the tip of the iceberg.

- In the journal Cell Host and Microbe—'*Control of Brain Development, Function and Behavior by the Microbiome*'[2]

- In the journal Microorganisms—'*The Gut Microbiome Feelings of the Brain: A Perspective for Non-Microbiologists*'[3]

- In the journal European Children and Adolescent Psychiatry—'*Gut microbiota and attention deficit hyperactivity disorder: new perspectives for a challenging condition*'[4]

- In the journal Frontiers of Neuroscience—'*Breaking down the barriers: the gut microbiome, intestinal permeability and stress-related psychiatric disorders*'[5]

- In the Journal of Alzheimer's Disease—'*Mechanisms of Molecular Mimicry Involving the Microbiota in Neurodegeneration*'[6]

- In the European Journal of Immunology—'*The role of the microbiota in inflammation, carcinogenesis and cancer therapy*'[7]

- In the World Journal of Gastroenterology—'*Influence of gut microbiota on neuropsychiatric disorders*'[8]

- In the British Medical Journal of Infectious Disease—'*Gut microbiota disturbance during helminth infection: can it affect cognition and behaviour of children?*'[9]

- In the journal Nature—'*Diet rapidly and reproducibly alters the human gut microbiome*'[10]

- In the journal Systems Biology in Medicine—'*The role of the microbiota in ageing: current state and perspectives*'[11]

- In the Journal of the American Heart Association—'*Intestinal Microbiota-Generated Metabolite Trimethylamine-N-Oxide and 5-Year Mortality Risk in Stable Coronary Artery Disease: The Contributory Role of Intestinal Microbiota in a COURAGE-Like Patient Cohort*'[12]

- In the journal Circulation Research—'*Gut microbiota-dependent trimethylamine N-oxide (TMAO) pathway contributes to both development of renal insufficiency and mortality risk in chronic kidney disease*'[13]

- In the Proceedings of the National Academy of Sciences—'Cross-talk between *Akkermansia muciniphila and intestinal epithelium controls diet-induced obesity*'[14]

Did that last one drop your jaw? Yes, it's true. Your microbiome controls whether or not you develop obesity from what you eat. Brain development in infants, generation of our emotions, neuropsychiatric disorders, ADHD, stress-related psychiatric disorders, Alzheimer's Disease, Parkinson's Disease, cancer, kids behavior, determining our health as we age and whether we're at risk of dying within 5 years from coronary artery disease—all are strongly determined by the microbiome. No system of the body is free from being directed (*hands on the steering wheel*) by the microbiome. No system of the body. That's how important the microbiome is.

When you really understand that the microbiome is driving your car, that it has its hands on the steering wheel of every system of your body, then it just makes sense that EVERY DAY we should put a small amount of attention in supporting the master regulating system of the body.

That's what you'll learn in this book—a routine to follow on a daily basis that's simple, easily adopted by the family and pretty much guarantees greater health and well-being.

And please don't feel threatened by this information. It takes most doctors years to change their paradigm and their thinking. We see articles every once in a while on the topic or we hear a presentation at a conference, reinforcing that this is an entire new world—and a critically important one. And they'll dip their toes in the water, occasionally telling a patient that it's a good idea to '*take a supplement of probiotics*' or '*eat a little yogurt for the good bacteria*'. That's what we knew back in the 80's and 90's. Now we know it's a much bigger picture than that. Supplements are beneficial. Homemade yogurts may be good for you. But the key to supporting the master regulator—which determines health and disease—is the diversity of the microbiome.

When I came into practice 40 years ago, we knew that if we prescribed probiotic supplements, many different conditions got better. And over the next four decades, more and more studies were published to validate and refine this observation. Hundreds and hundreds of studies. These studies validated all clinicians knowing that we were on the right track with 'shotgunning' in probiotic supplements for many different conditions. But in the last 15 years, with the Human Genome Project completed and technology allowing us to learn more and more about the body's composition (much more of *them* than us), we now know that it's the diversity of the microbiome, the thousands of different families of beneficial bacteria in our GI tract, that modulates our health or lack of health. And not just Lactobacillus or Bifidobacterium. They're important—but they're not the big picture.

Depending on the study you read, the number of Americans who are obese is about 33.7%. The number of Koreans (living in South Korea) that are obese is about 5.8% (remember the title of the last article above that I quoted to you on obesity). The US has 6 times the obesity that they have in South Korea. And it's not the sliders or the Big Macs or the french fries vs. the rice that they eat in South Korea. It's what your body does with the food that you eat. And who controls that? Yup—the microbiome. Koreans are born and raised into a culture that has a little bit of Kimchi each and every day. Constantly feeding the diversity of their microbiome.

This book is all about taking care of the primary modulator of your epigenome, the master control panel for all of the dimmer switches throughout your body—your microbiome—and how to build its healthy diversity. I have never seen a book for the general public as thorough, as easy to follow and as simple to implement as Dr. Susanne Bennett's *The Kimchi Diet*. And who better to learn from? Dr. Bennett is a 5th generation Natural Medicine Doctor born and raised in Korea (the motherland of building healthy microbiomes). She lives this concept of feeding the microbiome to build its diversity.

What do I think about this book? After reading it, I said to my wife, *"Honey, read this book. Then call Susanne. We're going to learn how to make kimchi. I want us to train our bodies (baby steps to begin with) to have a little kimchi every day."*

So, if I give a message like that to the person I love most in this life, how could I do any less for you? Read the book. Start what I'm calling the kimchi crawl (begin with baby steps, getting your gut used to kimchi). Learn more from Susanne in her online programs about this. And watch when a year from now your children's classmates are on another round of antibiotics from catching whatever is going around and you just smile, realizing that your kids have never been healthier.

Remember, *"base hits win the ballgame"*. This is a base hit that puts you and your family in the big leagues of vibrant health. Maybe even a double!

Towards healing the planet—one person at a time.

Dr. Tom O'Bryan

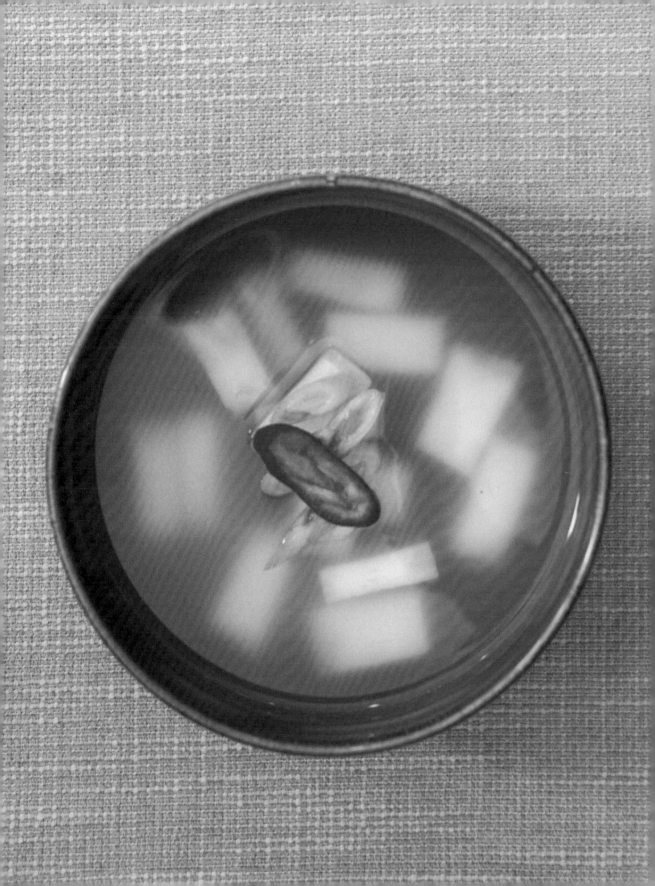

Introduction

Introduction

When the Severe Acute Respiratory Syndrome (SARS) virus hit Asia in 2003, it produced a global scare. The virus, with its terrible flu-like symptoms, often required intensive care and quickly spread to twenty-six countries and took over 700 lives before being contained a few months later. But one country in Asia was almost completely spared of the SARS epidemic—Korea. This puzzled scientists, but not Koreans, who quickly attributed their immunity to the country's national culinary treasure: kimchi. The *Los Angeles Times* reported that the consumption of kimchi began to spread in the months following the outbreak of SARS: "Southeast Asians are stocking up on it. China has embraced it. And South Koreans, who already eat it with every meal, are buying even more than usual."[1] This bit of folk wisdom about the healing powers of kimchi proved to be more than an urban legend. A 2010 animal study conducted in the aftermath of the outbreak revealed that:

> Tests and dissections conducted on chickens showed most birds that ate kimchi extract had no H1N1 bird flu or SARs viruses in their respiratory systems, while no mice that ate a special feed made from kimchi died in the experiment. The fatality rate for animals that were given regular feed, however, reached 20 percent.[2]

At the time, scientists had a host of theories about exactly *why* kimchi was so helpful. Was it the allicin in the garlic? The fiber-rich diet? The red pepper? Or was it the probiotic bacteria in kimchi itself? In fact, kimchi had so many healthful properties, it was difficult to isolate which *one* was contributing to its anti-SARS effects.

And while all of these factors might play a role, in 2018, a new study "concluded that bioactive compounds from lactic acid bacteria produced by kimchi fermentation serve as antiviral agents by affecting the virus membrane surface or promptly activating immune cells mobilization."[3] In other words, the helpful lactic acid bacteria (LAB) in fermented kimchi were attacking the viruses or helping to boost the immune system. Kimchi to the rescue!

The truth is, I wasn't the least bit surprised when I heard about kimchi's powers in fending off SARS. I was born in Seoul, Korea in the early sixties, on the heels of the Korean War. I attended the Seoul American Elementary School located on the Yongsan military base, where my father worked as a civilian for the U.S. government. We lived off-base, where the ambassadors' and diplomats' families resided, so I was exposed to a great deal of cultural diversity. My first language was Korean, and I didn't start speaking English until I began kindergarten at four years old.

For the first four years of my life, I ate like most other Koreans at the time. We had simple three-dish meals consisting of a soup, rice, and *banchan*, which were small

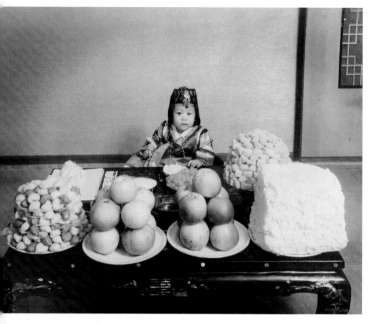

servings of seasonal vegetables and sometimes meat or seafood. And the number one banchan (side dish) that we ate pretty much every day at every meal, no matter what, was *kimchi*. To this day, most Koreans don't feel a meal is complete unless it comes with kimchi. Sometimes my mom would make radish kimchi, sometimes cabbage, and sometimes it was mustard greens. Other times my mother would use less common vegetables for something different. In the summertime, she'd make non-spicy versions of kimchi using vegetables like cucumbers. But no matter what, kimchi was there, day after day—an ancient, fermented superfood filled with vitamins, minerals, fiber, and probiotics.

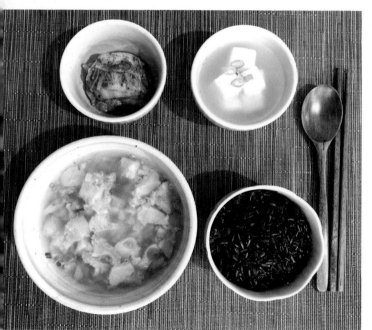

An ancient superfood that Western science has only now begun to catch up with.

So you can imagine my shock at four years old when I ate at the military base for the first time. Experiencing fast food was like going to Disneyland. It was a swirl of new flavors, smells, and textures. Every bite was so exciting: the aroma of fried foods and the richness of butter was divine. There were huge chunks of beef everywhere. And not to mention the ice cream, pies and other desserts!

But what my *body* remembers was that every time I ate cheeseburgers and french fries at the Officer's Club, something felt missing. I knew I wasn't getting something my body craved, something that was healthy and invigorating. All I wanted was to go home and have some kimchi. I think even then, intuitively, I knew deep in my gut that kimchi would be the best thing to settle a stomach bombarded with grease and fat. It's the best thing to help reset spiking blood sugar. Little did I know back then that it was the little friendly bacteria found in kimchi that my body was craving to heal my indigestion. Little did I know that kimchi was exactly the kind of fiber-rich, vitamin-rich food which was almost the exact opposite of everything I was eating at the base. Even then, I knew that there was something special about this wonder food, and that it cured so much of what was wrong with me when I would indulge in the typical American diet.

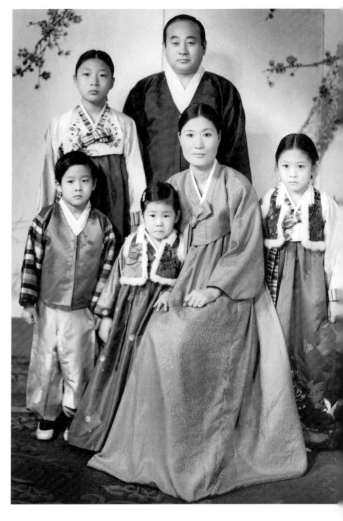

I was fortunate to grow up in an indigenous culture, but Korea at the time was also a third-world country where seated toilets and private showers were a luxury and sleeping elevated on a bed was only available to the U.S. military. Communal sleeping on the floor was the norm. But growing up in an indigenous culture also means that a great line of nutritional and health wisdom is passed down between generations, family to family, and especially mother to daughter. As a fifth-generation Korean traditional natural medicine doctor and someone who's also trained in Western medicine, I come from a long line of Koreans with a deep respect and appreciation for the healing properties of plants, both as food and as medicine. I've studied and experimented with herbs and plants for many years now to help settle stomachs, soothe rashes, relieve headaches and much more.

I couple my understanding of the healing role of food (given to me by my ancestors) with a scientific and biological knowledge of gut health, probiotics, and vitamin and mineral absorption in the body. I've had the chance to share what I know about the critical role diet plays in our modern epidemics in lectures and podcasts. I've also published books on allergy healing and prevention in *The 7-Day Allergy Makeover* and about mitochondrial health in *The Mighty Mito*. Over the past three decades, I've helped thousands of patients deal with chronic pain, obesity, low energy, allergies and more, often with simple but profound changes to diet and lifestyle. And you can bet that kimchi has often been a big part of all of this!

So why are fermented vegetables such a crucial part of Korean culture, and more importantly, how can kimchi revolutionize your health?

Kimchi—The World's Emerging Superfood

With the combination of thousands of years of cultural tradition behind it, and now

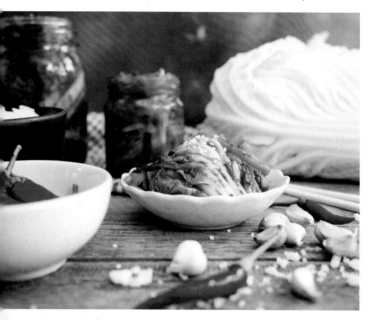

more and more scientific studies which validate its importance as one of the world's best functional foods, kimchi has attained a new popularity and recognition on the global stage. Kimchi flies off the shelves of grocery stores and appears on "Korean tacos" sold from taco trucks in Los Angeles and around the country. And its reputation is well deserved. As you'll learn in this book, researchers have linked kimchi consumption not just to its ability to help people fight off SARS, but to better overall immune response, gut health, weight loss, elevated mood and the prevention of a whole host of modern diseases, from diabetes to cancer to heart disease. There are a myriad of health reasons to eat kimchi, and I discuss them all in this book. In a country that has only recently caught on to the importance of probiotics and helpful gut bacteria, kimchi has thousands of years of cultivation and a complete nutritional profile, making it stand out even from sauerkraut, yogurt and other fermented foods.

Kimchi isn't just another food trend or fad. It's survived for thousands of years and best of all, it can be made by almost anyone, anywhere in the world.

Given my Korean heritage and lifelong love of kimchi, I

consider myself a "Kimchi Ambassador" to the world, sharing its virtues with my clients, on my website, and now to everyone reading this book. Kimchi isn't just another food trend or fad. It's survived for thousands of years and best of all, it can be made by almost anyone, anywhere in the world. Just think about it: what other superfood can you make with just a vegetable—*any* local vegetable—sea salt, garlic and ginger? You don't need fire, electricity, or gas to make kimchi. You don't need fancy kitchenware or rare ingredients. You just need a glass jar or a clay pot, some time, and the power of fermentation. It's truly a food that people across the globe in any economic circumstances can make and begin eating today to better their health and longevity. There's no reason that every American shouldn't be eating more of this wonder food, given our access to fresh, local, organic vegetables and how easy kimchi is to make.

Kimchi—Natural Cycles and Family Connection

But there's another lesson I think we can learn from this humble fermented vegetable.

One of my most sacred rituals has always been making kimchi with my family. Kimchi is related to the cycle of the seasons. The men often gather seafood to make paste in the spring and purchase the salt around this time. The family will harvest vegetables, such as radish or cabbage, in the fall. And together they'll make kimchi from scratch to mark the time of preparation for cold winter months. Kimchi and other fermented vegetables are what sustain you until the next spring.

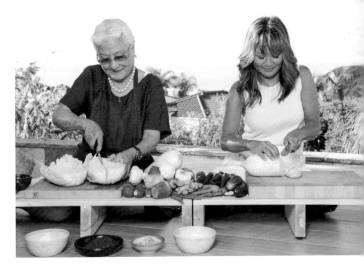

But it's not only about the natural cycles; kimchi is also about family. For me, there's no kimchi in the world better than my mother's. I have so many fond memories of her making it when I was a child. We lived high in the mountains where the temperature often dipped below freezing at night (winters in Korea are bitterly cold), but our kimchi was stored safely at the ideal temperature in earthenware pots, which were almost completely buried in the ground, with just the top edge of the pot and lid above ground. This meant that we were able to enjoy our kimchi all throughout the winter and spring, until fresh vegetables could be grown again, and turned into another batch of delicious kimchi in the summer.

Making kimchi is an affair that involves the whole family, particularly in the beginning of November, when my *eomeoni* (mother), *halmeoni* (grandmother), *emo* (aunt), and women in the neighborhood would gather at our home for *kimjang*, a yearly ritual that most Korean families participate in to make enough kimchi to last throughout the winter. Each year as winter approached, the family would harvest and gather a large crop of napa cabbage, radishes, carrots, and scallions, along with the necessary seasonings—mainly ginger, garlic and red pepper powder.

As the head of the household, Mom would plan out how many months of kimchi we would need to prepare so we'd have plenty of fermented vegetables to sustain us. Even though Korea is still considered a patriarchal society, it's the mother's responsibility to be in charge of *kimjang*. During this time in November, a new supply of fresh green vegetables might be six or seven months down the road, so it was important to make plenty of kimchi from the fall harvest: a huge responsibility that fell on the matriarch. Deciding what types of kimchi to prepare was also my mother's job—*baechu* (napa cabbage), *kkakdugi* (radish), *chongkak* (young radish) and *dongchimi* (radish water kimchi). Of course, it all depended on the availability of fresh vegetables and what we had that season. Although we had only six people in our family, we always had extended family and helpers at our home, so she needed to make enough kimchi for seven to nine people.

Once all of the vegetables were washed and brined with coarse sea salt for hours, my grandmother would make the special kimchi sauce, a recipe that's been passed down from generation to generation. Once the kimchi was in the ground, it only needed to ferment for a few days before we could start to enjoy it, but it tasted even better after a few weeks. The flavor and texture would change as time went on and it continued to slowly ferment while buried in the ground. It started off mild and crunchy, and as time went on, the flavors became much more complex and the texture of the vegetables would soften quite a bit. Before long, we had a delicious, nutritious treat that got us through the cold months. And we did it together—as a family.

I hope that as part of reading this book and experimenting with the recipes, you take time to make kimchi a family affair as well. There's almost nothing more bonding, more fun, and more wonderful than making a delicious meal together as a family. And kimchi is one of the healthiest foods you can offer your family.

What Inspired This Book

As a physician, my real passion and interest in kimchi and *kimchiology* (the science of kimchi and the kimchi microbiome) began in 2013 when I went back to visit my birth place for the first time after leaving in 1975. Naturally, we went to all of the tourist attractions in various parts of South Korea, and the "K-food" culture was amazing!

What struck me was the enormous amount of carbohydrates that Korean people ate: hundreds and hundreds of grams of carbohydrates at every meal—including white rice, wheat-based noodles and sweet pastries made from all types of flour. What was even more dumbfounding was that these people were not overweight at all. In fact, I barely saw any overweight children or adults, both in big cities and in the countryside. Interestingly, the obesity rate of South Korea is only at 5.8%, whereas in the United States the obesity rate is at 33.7% with over 73.8 million obese people. We're in first place in the US, with the highest number of obese people in one country. Furthermore, the Koreans I saw were all very energetic and physically fit with vibrant, clear skin. In appearance, Korean people looked extremely healthy.

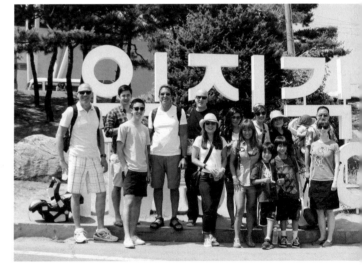

So it led me to wonder: what was so different in Korea compared to the United States? Why could Koreans eat five to ten times as many carbs as Americans but not suffer the seemingly bad effects? Why had the obesity epidemic and all the negative health consequences that go with it like inflammation, diabetes, and heart issues not struck the Korean peninsula?

By the end of my family vacation and after observing thousands of people at restaurants, festivals and street food culture, I came to the conclusion that there was only one major factor that was *clearly* different between the Korean and western diet. The secret wasn't in the main courses, but in the side dish Koreans ate at every meal. The fermented, probiotic-dense side dish they ate even with burgers and pizza.

And that was kimchi.

As soon as I got back, I started incorporating kimchi into every one of my patients' dietary protocols. And for the past five years, working with thousands of acute and chronic illnesses, I've had the chance to learn from trial and error which kimchi works best for specific symptoms and issues. I've discovered the fastest ways to use kimchi to

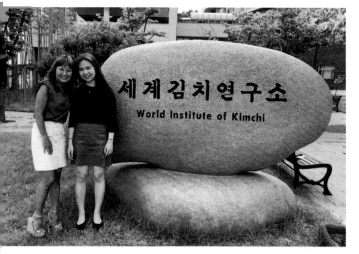

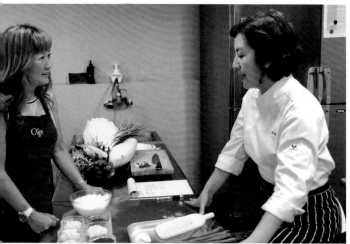

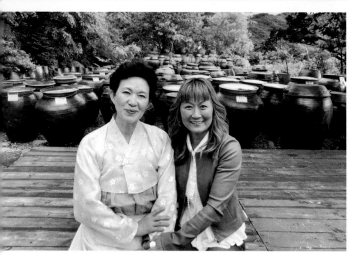

heal the gut, reduce inflammation, clear up acne, help with mood, and so much more. There was a consistent pattern that developed and eventually I came up with "The Kimchi Diet™." With most diets, you're asked to eliminate foods. But with The Kimchi Diet™, it's all about adding a simple fermented side dish to improve your health. After my trip to my homeland and seeing so many of my patients experience amazing results with The Kimchi Diet™, I was first inspired to write this book.

But I needed to learn even more. I started to read everything there was to know about kimchi before writing. I also went back to South Korea, where it all started. Going on a self-funded research trip was truly one of the best experiences of my life. I got to dig deeper into my heritage and talk to many Korean people in the kimchi industry. I rode a bullet train going over 200 miles per hour down to Gwangju to visit and videotape the Kimchi Museum. I was very fortunate to speak to the experts at the World Institute of Kimchi (WIKIM), a one-of-a-kind research facility where the scientists' sole purpose is to study the science of kimchi, its microbiome, and its effects on the human body. In fact, the word *kimchiology* was coined by WIKIM. I also had a private kimchi-making lesson with the CEO and founder of O'ngo Foods, Dr. Jia Choi, where I learned a couple of new tips on kimchi that improved my recipes. Visiting one of the few organically certified red pepper farms was truly enlightening as well, seeing how its greenhouses were meticulously clean, free of pests, air pollution, and cross-contamination from other farms. The highlight of my trip was visiting the Bori Kimchi Farm, where I got to interview the most famous Kimchi Masterchef, Ha Yeon Lee. You can watch a series of videos of my trip online. Check out the Resource section on page 153 for the link.

During my trip, I started getting amazing ideas on what I'd like to add to the book, and had a deep realization when I was hiking up Namsan Mountain, where my house was once located. I realized that I was completing a trilogy of books that began with *The 7-Day Allergy Makeover* and led into *Mighty Mito*. In my first book, I tell the story of my lifelong quest to understand allergies after my son, Cody was born with debilitating and life-threatening allergies that required numerous hospital visits each year. I trace out a plan of diet, lifestyle, and emotional changes that anyone can implement to help their body better deal with allergens. The book is based on my clinical work, research, and private practice since 1996.

And allergens are all around us in this modern world. So rather than just focus only on the obvious sources of allergens—pollen, pet dander, and dust mites—the book takes a broad view of allergies, showing how exposure to volatile organic compounds, pesticides, gluten, dairy and environmental toxicants can create a host of symptoms, from sluggishness and brain fog to decreased immune response and inflammation. I explain that allergies aren't just about sneezing or anaphylactic (IgE) reactions, but about the burden of a toxic load of allergens harming our most vital functions and taking a toll on our bodies day after day.

In *The Mighty Mito*, I tell the story of how I recovered from a brain injury after I slammed my head into an open refrigerator door above me. Despite having tried many medical and alternative therapies, nothing worked until I focused on mitochondrial recovery. Mitochondria are the powerhouses of the cell, the place where energy in the form of adenosine triphosphate (ATP) is produced. The more mitochondria are unable to function properly—and a brain injury can severely limit them—the less energy the body has to deal with other problems. Intense neck pain, rapid muscle loss, anxiety, insomnia, and problems with memory and cognitive function were my daily lot. By creating a diet plan, including my own mitochondrial superfood—oxygenated pudding—taking key supplements, and working on specific kinds of exercise and stress reduction, I was able to heal what so many acupuncturists, chiropractors, and even medical doctors had not been able to. I was focused on giving my cells more oxygen, lowering the amount of free radicals in my system (avoiding harmful pollutants and processed foods), doing targeting exercises, and staying away from the sugars that used *anaerobic* (non-oxygen based) processes to produce energy.

Soon, however, I realized the plan I created was not just good for treating my own brain injury, but a protocol that could help others to heal from a litany of diseases by revving up the energy-producing capacities of the body's mighty mitochondria. A body's true biological age can be measured by the amount of cellular damage, and the more we nurture our mitochondria, the younger we can look and feel.

So how does all of this connect to kimchi? I realized in each of these books that I'm telling a story of women—of the biological and cultural legacies passed on to us by women, of mothers and daughters, mothers and sons, and how women shape our genes, internal biomes, and bodies. Let me explain.

In *The 7-Day Allergy Makeover*, I reveal that one of the root causes of Cody's allergies was triggered by something that happened while he was in my womb. I had mercury tooth fillings at the time, and they started to leach toxic mercury into my body and eventually into my breast milk. Even as a six-month old, he was battling the toxicity of mercury in his system, not to mention other allergens like eggs, dairy, gluten, mold, nuts, and more.

And since Cody was a C-section baby, he didn't get exposed to my natural flora as he would have if he'd been born the traditional way through the birth canal. He was cheated out of the most important inoculation of his life, one that would steer his immune system on the right path. This experience made me realize just how intimately linked a mother's health and microbiome are to what she passes on to her children in terms of native flora and immune health.

In addition, it made me realize how the more allergens and toxicants we ingest, the more we pass those on to our children while they're in the womb and during breastfeeding. It also started my quest into understanding gut health and gut bacteria, which has culminated in this book. Mothers in a very real sense *create* the biological realities of their children's bodies, and in a way they're responsible for their children's ability to adapt and for their epigenetic expressions.

Our mitochondrial DNA (mtDNA) is 100% maternally inherited. As I explained in *Mighty Mito*, epigenetic changes to mtDNA, that is, changes that take place during a person's life, including mutations and damage, greatly impact their overall health. So just as a mother's exposure to toxicants and allergens can shape a child's early development and biological constitution, so too her exposure to oxidative stress, free radicals, and the damage they cause to mitochondria also gets passed down maternally. All the more important for women who choose to have children to take care of their bodies before, during and after pregnancy.

Finally, when it comes to kimchi, I'm writing the story of a female tradition—of kimchi being passed from grandmother to mother to daughter, across hundreds or even thousands of years. But it's more than that. Western medicine is only now catching on to the vital importance of our gut biome—the bacteria and microbial flora in our stomach and intestines—to our overall health. And is it any surprise that our gut biome is shaped by and inherited from our mothers? When we're born, we receive our first dose of microbial inoculation from our mother via the birth canal. This native flora sets us up for healthy gut flora of our own for life. And one of the best ways for a mother to get a healthy gut microbiome is to eat fermented foods over the years. From there, the food that we eat dictates the type and amounts of different bacteria that thrive in and on our body, choices that in many cultures are shaped predominantly by mothers. Kimchi, this fermented wonder food, is one of the single best things a mother can eat to create a healthy gut biome, and "pass down" her flora to her children, and continuing through the female lineage, generation after generation. *The Kimchi Diet* is the last book of the trilogy, creating the full circle of life!

The Benefits of Kimchi: A Brief Overview

One gram of kimchi gives you, on average, *one billion* probiotic organisms. Probiotic pills often have about five billion, perhaps up to ten billion. So how big is one gram of kimchi? Think of it this way: 4.2 grams is just one *teaspoon.* If you eat my suggested ½ cup per day, you'll get 100 billion CFUs of lactic acid bacteria daily. And the average Korean used to eat about 300 grams of kimchi per day, before Westernization. In other words, they'd resupply their system with 300 billion probiotic organisms per day! That's right—instead of taking expensive probiotic pills, you can get all of the health benefits and more from eating kimchi. Another great thing about kimchi is that you're not just getting five or six strains, but close to a thousand different strains of probiotics, all of which can help to fight pathogenic bacteria and perform different functions in the body.

And it's become very clear just how important it is to cultivate beneficial microbes in our gut. Having an unhealthy gut biome has been linked to issues such as irritable bowel syndrome, (including constipation and bloating)[4] as well as cardiovascular disease and CDI or *clostridium difficile* infection.[5] Not only that, but there's more research than ever pointing to the vagus nerve as a connector between the gut and the brain and its role in "interoceptive" awareness, a sense of what's going on with our gut microbes.[6] So metaphors about "feeling it in my gut" or having a "gut sense" may turn out to be far more than just metaphors. Scientists call this "gut-brain" the *enteric nervous system*, a counterpart for the one that runs through our brain. And when there are problems in the gut, there can be problems with anxiety and depression.

This has fueled the probiotics craze. And while many foods are now eager to boast about their "probiotic" potential, the side effects of these foods—the sugars, wheat or dairy that often go into them—sometimes offsets any benefits for the biome due to the inflammatory or allergic reactions they induce. Real kimchi, however, is dairy-free, gluten-free, raw, predigested and loaded with probiotics. Not only are you helping your gut, you're getting a heavy dose of vitamins, minerals, fiber and antioxidants along the way. As you'll read about in Chapter 2, the science also shows kimchi consumption has been linked to weight loss, improved immunity, lower inflammation, clearer skin, heart health, cancer prevention and so much more.

What You'll Find in This Book

Kimchi is the universal superfood: it can be added to any diet, from keto to paleo to vegan to kosher to Mediterranean.

I believe the fastest way to improve chronic symptoms is to change what you eat, and adding kimchi to your diet is the fastest and best way to improve your nutrition. If you're suffering from acne, eczema, gas and bloating, difficulty losing weight, or muscle and joint aches, this book is for you. Likewise, if you're concerned about long term issues like heart health, cancer prevention and staying happy and fit, you'll find out exactly why incorporating kimchi into your diet is one of the best things you can do.

This book is divided into five chapters and offers an overview of kimchi, shows you how to make it, explains its health benefits, and gives you an 8-week plan for creating enough kimchi to feed your family and begin a new healthy way of eating that incorporates this fermented treat. Best of all, kimchi is the universal superfood: it can be added to any diet, from keto to paleo to vegan to kosher to Mediterranean.

In chapter 1, I offer a brief history of kimchi, its role in Korean society, and how it attained its current global status as one of the best superfoods around. I also discuss other fermented foods and explain what sets kimchi apart from the rest.

Chapter 2 details the scientific studies that have linked increased kimchi consumption and probiotics to weight loss, better immunity, lower inflammation, clearer skin, improved mood, cancer prevention, and a host of other health benefits.

In chapter 3, I lay out the 8-week plan for making and consuming kimchi, including an overview of the anti-inflammatory diet that I recommend all of my patients eat for maximum results. While eating kimchi alone can make you feel better, coupling it with an overall plan for healthful eating is really the way to go.

Chapter 4 goes into how to brine, prepare, and store kimchi and includes my best kimchi-making tips.

In chapter 5, recipes that I've been handed down and refined over the years will be given to you to put to use. Once you make your first batch of kimchi and get the hang of it, you'll see that the recipes are easy to follow, quick to make, and so tasty! I'm sure you'll be eager to jump right in and start making kimchi regularly, passing up on the commercially made ones!

A Final Word

Even though I've lived in the U.S. for several decades now, I still love and crave kimchi and eat it daily, not just for the delicious mouthwatering taste, but for its medicinal properties. Every time I come back from a medical conference, where organic food is non-existent, the first food I grab is a half-cup of kimchi. When I get a big dose of radiation from going through airport security, kimchi calms my spirit and gets me back on track. If I get a bad

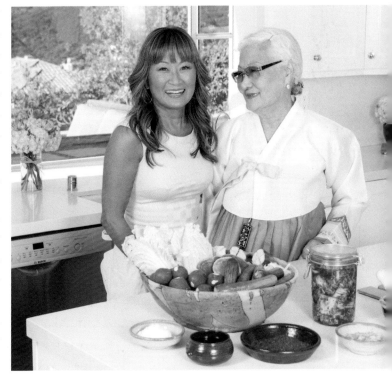

case of food poisoning or have diarrhea, I go for the kimchi juice cure instead of commercial stomach relievers. If I ever have constipation, a cup of kimchi is the best natural laxative. I think you'll soon discover that kimchi remedies are endless.

That's why I've dedicated this book to my wonderful mother, who's always put as much love into her kimchi as any other ingredient. My aim is to help familiarize you with all the wonders and benefits of kimchi, so that you'll start enjoying it as a regular part of your diet today and every day!

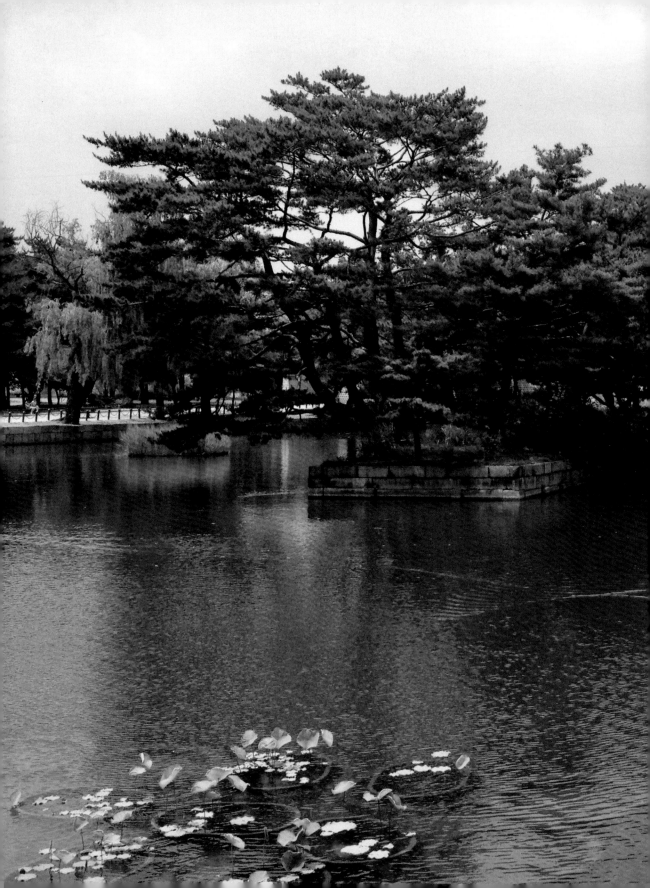

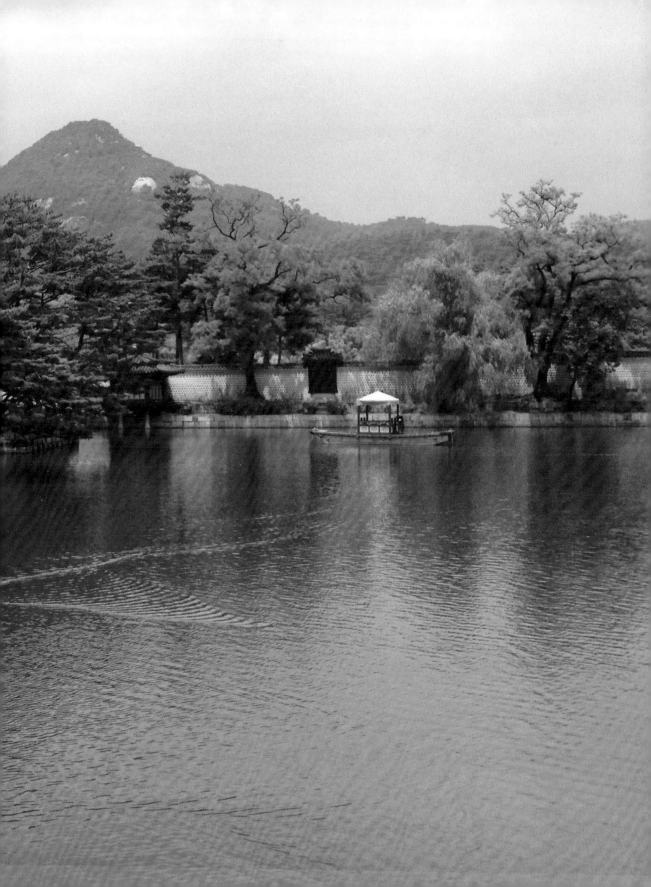

Chapter 1

History of Kimchi

You might not think that kimchi—this simple dish of salted and fermented vegetables—can revolutionize your health. But it's one of the great superfoods of the modern world and according to *Health Magazine*, one of the healthiest things you can eat, anywhere on the planet. *UNESCO* (the United Nations Educational Scientific and Cultural Organization) recently recognized *kimjang* or the practice of winter-time kimchi preparation as part of the "intangible heritage" of humanity. As their website says, making kimchi provides an "opportunity for strengthening family cooperation" and reminds us that "human communities need to live in harmony with nature."[1] This lofty designation might sound like a lot to live up to, but I believe that kimchi—its preparation, its connection to natural cycles of the earth, and of course, all its health benefits—has a lot to teach our modern world.

In a world overrun by obesity, diabetes, and heart disease, you'll be happy to know that kimchi consumption has been linked to weight loss, better immunity, superior digestion, improved colon health, and lower blood pressure. It's low in calories, high in fiber, full of antioxidants, vitamins A and C, and as a fermented food, packed with probiotics, those helpful bacteria that improve our gut functioning. It's a surprise that in this day and age of health foods going mainstream, more people aren't taking advantage of all kimchi's benefits by rushing out and buying more. Or better yet, creating their own.

In a world overrun by obesity, diabetes, and heart disease, you'll be happy to know that kimchi consumption has been linked to weight loss, better immunity, superior digestion, improved colon health, and lower blood pressure.

This book is here to change that. I'm going to share with you the secrets of this magical Korean food and give you a complete plan to make it, preserve it and integrate it into your diet, so you too can enjoy all these health benefits. Not to mention the delicious taste!

So why hasn't it caught on sooner? The truth is, kimchi has only recently (within the last 50–60 years) been introduced to the West, and outside of a few major centers like New York and Los Angeles (where I live), Korean food until recently hasn't caught on the way that Thai food or Indian food did in earlier decades. Furthermore, it's only within the last five to ten years that the amazing powers of kimchi have caught the attention of scientists and researchers in this country. Meanwhile, Koreans—as well as their neighbours in China and Japan—have known about the value of this amazing pickled food for hundreds of years, and it's cited time after time by the Koreans I spoke with as a leading factor in helping them live longer, healthier and happier lives. But as research on probiotics, raw and living foods, antioxidants, and plant-based diets has grown in the last decade, more and more scientists have come to see kimchi as the perfect embodiment of all of these converging health trends.

The other reason it may not have caught on fully yet is that many in the West have been turned off by its reputation for being "too spicy" or "too pungent" in its fermentation. However, this reputation is often unfairly founded only on mass-produced, commercialized, store-bought brands of napa cabbage kimchi which are soaked in red pepper powder. This is not to say that all store-bought forms of kimchi are bad, but they don't represent the great diversity and complexity of kimchi in Korea. Many kinds of kimchi don't use red pepper. Many kinds of kimchi are fermented for far shorter periods of time than others, resulting in a less pronounced "fermented" taste. Likewise, for those people who aren't fans of cabbage (I personally find it delicious), you'll be happy to know you can make kimchi not only from carrots, radishes, and cucumbers, but also from more exotic foods like watermelons and jicama. Check the Resource section on page 153 to get bonus kimchi recipes online.

And if you already love kimchi, but have only tried what's for sale in most health food or Asian grocery stores, you're in for quite a treat!

So it makes sense to start with a short history of kimchi: how it came to be developed, its role in Korean culture, how it's become part of the industrialized, modern world, and why returning to the traditional ways of making kimchi that I'm going to share with you in this book is the best way to optimize its full potential.

Kimchi Origins

No one knows exactly when kimchi was created, but we do know that it goes back at least several thousand years to Korea's "Three Kingdoms" period between 57 BCE and 668 CE. The early Korean diet consisted of meat, seafood and an assortment of berries, roots and vegetables. Pots were used between 6,000 and 3,000 BCE to store fish and vegetables, making researchers believe that the first cases of fermentation on the Korean peninsula began around this time, as foods would have naturally fermented and been beneficial to eat due to their superior nutritional and probiotic content. Conscious storing of vegetables and seafood protected them from hot summers and the harsh winter conditions prominent on the peninsula. People in Korea cultivated various vegetables and grains such as millet and rice—and eventually soybeans. Soybeans were fermented even before the creation of kimchi, and this process eventually led to the development of dishes such as *bulgogi* (meat marinated in fermented soybean sauce) and traditional Korean seasonings such as *doenjang* (fermented soybean paste), or, when combined with red pepper, the now world-famous *gochujang* hot paste. However, kimchi proper only developed somewhere between 100 BCE and 600 CE. It rose to prominence as more Koreans became Buddhist, a religion that emphasizes nonviolence toward living creatures and hence, a vegetarian diet.

Early versions of kimchi (Kingdom Kimchi) were quite different from most of today's recipes due to availability or lack of certain vegetables and seasonings throughout the year. Early kimchi often consisted of radishes fermented in a salt paste or brine, since Chinese cabbage (aka "napa" or "kimchi" cabbage) wasn't popular in Korea until several hundred years later. This version of kimchi wasn't spicy at all, as red pepper (*gochu*) wasn't yet available in Korea. Today most people's idea of kimchi is the version called *baechu-kimchi*, which you can find in almost every Korean's home. It's made with napa cabbage, Korean radish, *gochugaru* (red pepper powder), and various seasonings like garlic, ginger and scallions. Sometimes fermented seafood (*jeotgal*) is also included in the seasoning mix, especially in the coastal regions of Korea.

There are conflicting theories as to when red pepper (a critical ingredient in most kimchi recipes today) was first introduced in Korea. The popular belief is that red pepper was introduced by Japan in the 16th century, and this is what is taught in schools and written in various texts in Japan. However, many Koreans disagree with this theory, and historical writings from Korea's Three Kingdoms period from more than a 1,000 years earlier indicate that red pepper (or at least a similar type of plant) was cultivated for use in kimchi recipes during that period.[2] Either way, we're certainly grateful for red pepper's wide availability around the world now, as it provides a unique, warm and spicy flavor that many Koreans can't imagine living without.

For at least the last century, the typical Korean meal has consisted of rice (*bap*), soup (*kuk*) and some kind of kimchi—along with several different side dishes known as *banchan*. These *banchan* are typically marinated vegetables such as bean sprouts, bellflower, gobo root and radish—but it's safe to say that no Korean meal is complete without a serving of kimchi. This traditional diet allowed Koreans to get carbohydrates from rice, protein and fat from animal broth and meat (often fish) in their soups—if they were not vegetarian—and vitamins and minerals, as well as helpful probiotics from kimchi, even in winter. Along with that, the typical Korean diet stressed fish over red meat, lots of legumes like soybeans, medicinal herbs, no processed or deep-fried foods, and was the original farm-to-table, local and seasonal cuisine. Traditionally, Korean meals are served all at once, with all the food on the table, making them a true sight for the eyes, with their array of textures and colors. Hopefully you can see why this type of diet has survived for millennia and continues to be eaten by people across the Korean peninsula to this day, which should be an inspiration for our own eating habits in whatever country we live in.

Kimjang and Regional Varieties of Kimchi

The origins of kimchi-making go back to a tradition known as *kimjang*, as mentioned above, a one-month period in part of November and December during which tens of thousands of households across Korea prepare their surplus from the autumn harvest for storage over winter. During colder times, when vegetables were not plentiful, kimchi became one of the only sources of essential vitamins and minerals for ancient Koreans. But the necessary steps for kimjang begin months before. Springtime was when seafood was purchased. Sea salt was bought in summer, and fall was when the vegetables ripened for harvest. Kimjang required the whole society to get on board, just as the entire household was involved. The husband would have to spend money for the cabbages, radishes, garlic, seafood, ginger, or scallions that his family didn't produce on their own. Wives were in charge of the preparation of the food: washing, chopping, salting and storing the vegetables

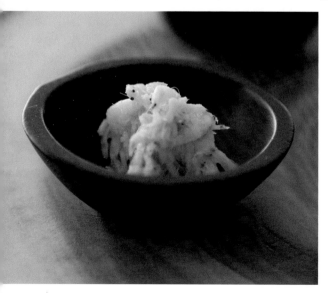

for the winter. Traditionally, kimchi was stored in earthenware clay storage pots and put underground throughout the winter months. The process involved not just each family, but the community as a whole, which would work together, celebrate together, and often share kimchi varieties with their friends and relatives. Each region and even each village would produce a different kind of kimchi, based on different lengths of fermentation, saltiness, spice level, and of course, the vegetables used.

For this reason, each region in Korea has become known for distinct types of kimchi that persist to this day. For instance, Gangwon-do uses less salted seafood, *jeotgal*, whereas Hamgyeong-do to the north incorporates squid, flatfish, and pollock. Pyeongan-do is known for more watery and mild kimchis, like its neighbor Hwanghae-do, which also has a more neutral taste, lacking the red pepper powder so prominent in most mass market kimchi. Gyeongsang-so in the southeast has some of the spiciest and saltiest kimchi—it's really a place for those who love extremes, as is its neighbor Jeolla-do to the west, with its incorporation of fermented seafood and red pepper.

With over 250 types of kimchi, each region of Korea is known for its specialities, just as in the United States one might argue not only argue about the merits of deep-dish Chicago pizza versus New York pizza, but also the use of totally different ingredients on it, such as pineapple, sun-dried tomatoes, or barbecued chicken! After World War II and the coming of mass production, these regional differences have lost some of their meaning. But the traditional ways of making kimchi do not disappear overnight. The regions still retain some of their characteristic ways of making, salting, and spicing kimchi, and this is especially true of rural people who continue to make kimchi in the traditional ways.

Kimchi Variations

What are some of the 250 kinds of kimchi that Korea has produced over the years? First, when most people hear the word *kimchi*, they likely think of the spicy fermented napa cabbage dish known as *baechu-kimchi*, but there are actually many kimchi recipes which aren't spicy and that don't even include cabbage. In fact, baechu-kimchi may be a far more recent addition to the Korean repertoire, with radishes, open-leafed cabbages, scallions, fish, and even grains preceding the use of napa cabbage.

As mentioned above, the vegetables and seasonings used in kimchi preparations throughout history depended heavily on what was available seasonally in each region of Korea. In the coastal regions, fermented salted seafood (jeotgal) such as shrimp, fish, clams, and oysters is commonly used for flavoring. In the more inland areas, different vegetables and seasonings were used, depending on what could be grown locally each season.

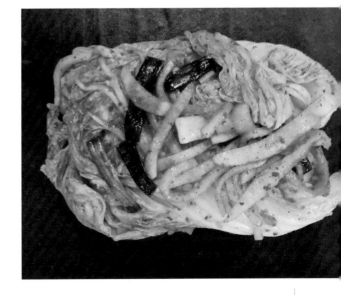

A common misconception is that kimchi is always fermented. And although it's arguably most tasty and addictive when fermented for anywhere from a few days to a few months, it's commonly consumed fresh as well, especially in the summer. Fresh unfermented kimchi made with cabbage is called *baechu-geotjeori*, but it can also be made fresh with other vegetables like cucumbers and Korean radishes.

Dongchimi (radish water kimchi) is usually made with fresh radishes right before winter starts and is fermented with the usual kimchi seasonings. The flavor and texture of dongchimi is quite different from cabbage kimchi, and everyone has their own preference, but I adore them both equally. Check the Resource section for my dongchimi recipe on page 153!

Gam kimchi uses persimmons, radish, and cabbage. So yes, even fruits can be turned into kimchi! And for those who love Halloween, you'll be glad to know that pumpkins can be made into kimchi in what's known as *hobak kimchi*.

Another favorite is *oi kimchi*, which I think almost anyone who has never had kimchi will love. It's made with cucumbers instead of napa cabbage or radishes and is the first kimchi I recommend everyone to start with while on The Kimchi Diet™ plan. Oi kimchi can be eaten fresh or fermented and is a wonderfully refreshing summer kimchi.

Nabak kimchi, or water kimchi, is often made and enjoyed in the warm summer months. It contains much more salty brine than other kimchi recipes. The flavorful broth

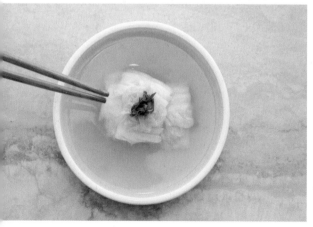

can be ladled over rice or noodles, used as a soup base or drunk straight as a crisp thirst-quencher. These simpler kimchis were often made throughout the warmer months and didn't involve as much effort as those made during the harsh winter months of *kimjang*.

In Chapter 5 of this book (page 127), you'll find my Kimchi Diet™ Recipes for each phase of the program, including the cucumber kimchi, to get you started on the right path to better health!

Kimchi Today

Nowadays, eating kimchi is a delightful and rich experience for the palate, combining sweet, tart, salty, and *umami* flavors (umami is the most recently discovered taste, translated from Japanese it means savory and delicious). In the most basic terms, "kimchi" is simply the Korean word for "fermented vegetables." These days, it's usually made by fermenting napa cabbage or radishes. But it can be made with virtually any type of vegetable, and even some fruits. It can be made with or without red peppers or other seasonings. What makes it especially healthful is the one-two punch of super nutritious veggies combined with the magical properties of probiotics, the helpful gut bacteria found in fermented foods like yogurt, sauerkraut, and kefir. In Chapter 2, we'll go deeper into its many health benefits.

The popularity of kimchi has spread far and wide in the past century and it's now consumed in many countries around the world in large amounts. Koreans eat on average about 40–50 pounds of kimchi a year, with 63% of it still being made at home.[3] Many neighboring countries either import kimchi from Korea or make their own, including for export. Japan for instance accounts for about 80% of Korea's exports of kimchi, while much of the kimchi consumed in Korea is now made at a low cost in China, a result of industrialization and mass production. I prefer kimchi made in Korea, as it tends not only to taste better but generally isn't made with food additives or chemicals. In the United States, you can find kimchi in most health food stores, Asian markets and even a few traditional supermarkets. But be on the lookout for additives and chemicals, even in many seemingly "healthy" kimchi packages.

Koreans eat on average about 40–50 pounds of kimchi a year, with 63% of it still being made at home.

Before industrialization, fermented foods were much more commonly consumed than they are today, which is unfortunate because they're still an excellent way to preserve food for long periods of time without the need for refrigeration. They're tough to beat when it comes to nutrition and their positive effects on gut health. However, with the rise of refrigeration, it's now possible to keep vegetables fresher for longer. The unfortunate side effect is that before refrigeration was widely available, people around the world had to find the most effective ways to keep their food fresh for as long as possible. Fermentation was always one of the most popular ways to accomplish this task. This food preservation method was used for everything from bread to alcohol to fruits and vegetables to dairy products—and just about every other type of food imaginable, bringing with it a host of health benefits that a refrigerator can't duplicate.

In today's busy world, where convenience is king, many Koreans and others around the globe are choosing to buy kimchi and other fermented foods at the grocery store rather than making their own. Many of the store-bought varieties have added MSG or other artificial sweeteners and chemicals. But store-bought kimchi can still confer a host of nutritional benefit from consuming it, so long as it's all-natural, non-pasteurized, and remains as close to homemade kimchi as possible.

The Process of Fermentation

For thousands of years, people around the globe have been fermenting all kinds of food and beverages. Each culture has developed its unique ways of producing and storing its precious creations, from clay pots to modern airtight containers. If you aren't familiar with how fermented foods are made, here's a quick primer.

The fermentation of food is a natural process that takes place in an anaerobic (oxygen-free) environment, where yeasts and bacteria (including multiple strains of lactic acid bacteria, or LAB) which are naturally present on the food convert starches and sugars in the foods into various acids and alcohols. Vegetables are usually fermented in a salt brine (salt and water mixture) or a salty paste in order to inhibit any harmful molds or unwanted bacteria from growing. Salt allows lactic acid bacteria to grow and multiply, but it kills off virtually all harmful bacteria in fermented food, such as E. Coli. Good bacteria feed off the vegetables (and other food used), release acids and gases, and preserve the food for us. When we eat the food, we get both the great nutrition *and* ingest these beneficial lactic acid bacteria.

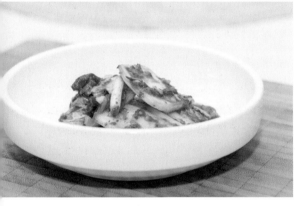

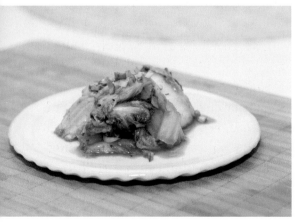

The fermentation process usually takes anywhere from a day or two up to a few months, depending on the type of fermented food, the ambient temperature, and how ripe or sour you prefer it to taste. Once it's sufficiently fermented, the food is usually stored in a cool place like the fridge, a cellar or in the ground (depending on the season and part of the world). This slows down the fermentation process dramatically, so that you can enjoy the food before it becomes too sour or too mushy. Traditionally, many cultures have fermented vegetables in order to have a store of them for the winter months. Instead of letting the excess of the autumn harvest go to waste, people figured out an ingenious way to enjoy vegetables through the dark days of December, January and February (in the northern hemisphere, that is). Not only did they prevent spoilage, but they created some of the world's first superfoods, loaded with beneficial probiotic bacteria. These "friendly" bacteria are incredibly helpful in maintaining optimal digestion, immune function and so much more.

Humankind has had a long and intimate relationship with the microbes that are present in our food, even before we realized they existed. For countless centuries, we've fermented food in order to extend the shelf life of our harvest, to make food more palatable (some food tastes much better fermented than raw, like cabbage) and because we've found these foods to be of great nutritional and medicinal value.

Humankind has had a long and intimate relationship with the microbes that are present in our food, even before we realized they existed.

Fermented Foods Around the World

Flavorful kimchi is Korea's most notable contribution to the world of fermented food, but Korea is also known for its fermented soybean paste and soy sauce (which originated in Korea), fermented red pepper powder paste and fermented fish, just to name a few of its other delicious creations. While this book focuses on kimchi, I wanted to share some of the other foods that you may wish to consider if you want to get all you can out of the world's array of fermented dishes and the helpful probiotics found in them.

Yogurt

In the United States, yogurt is the most popular cultured food, and probably the one that most people eat on a regular basis. Although there's no clear proof, many experts believe that yogurt was invented in the Middle East over 7,000 years ago. Nowadays, you can find dozens of types of yogurt, from blueberry and strawberry to Greek yogurt to dairy-free coconut yogurt. Unfortunately, traditional milk-based yogurt is one of the fermented foods I'm least likely to recommend to those seeking my nutritional advice. The truth is, most of the yogurt found in grocery stores have been made with pasteurized milk, which can affect the level of beneficial bacteria you're hoping to ingest. Plus, it often contains lots of sugar and other additives, which results in low lactic acid bacteria counts. By reintroducing sugar or fake chemicals, companies are actually destroying the health benefits that traditionally made yogurts *do* have. This is true even of many supposedly "healthy" yogurts like ones based in non-dairy milks. Beyond this tendency toward added sugars, yogurt causes digestive problems for many people. A good number of people—many without knowing it—are intolerant of or sensitive to dairy. They may experience symptoms like extreme bloating, gas, constipation or diarrhea. Some develop skin issues, such as acne or eczema. I personally advise choosing plant-based milk yogurts made of almond, coconut, or rice. Make sure that they're *not* pasteurized, as well. Coconut or almond yogurt are probably the best options if you decide to go this route.

Pickles

Pickles are made from cucumbers fermented in a salty brine (sometimes with garlic or other seasonings added) and are possibly the second-most popular of fermented foods eaten in the United States. They're crunchy, tangy and refreshing, and the Kosher Dills that are so abundant in supermarkets today were enjoyed for centuries by Jewish people living in Eastern Europe. When immigrants from this region came to the United States, they brought their pickling practices with them, making pickles a staple on all kinds of sandwiches and burgers.

Pickles are super quick and easy to make and are a smart way to preserve an overabundance of cucumbers that you may be faced with at the end of summer if you have a vegetable garden. Unfortunately, like yogurt, most of the pickles that you'll find in grocery stores these days have been pasteurized, so they've lost their probiotics and live enzymes. Or they've been preserved in a vinegar base instead of being fermented in a salt brine. However, fermenting and preserving your own pickles is a great practice and will allow you to enjoy all the health benefits of the lactic acid bacteria they contain. Koreans have a cucumber kimchi which uses cut-up cucumbers and is light and refreshing for the summer, and often made without spicy red pepper.

Sourdough Bread

Sourdough is another favorite around the world, and it's believed to have originated in ancient Egypt thousands of years ago. Before baker's yeast was created in the last century, sourdough was *the* method for leavening breads of all sorts, and this ancient method is still used today all over the globe. Sourdough bread is higher in nutrients, easier to digest and has a much more complex flavor than bread made with commercial yeast. As with pickles, European immigrants who emigrated to America in the 1800's brought their precious sourdough starter culture with them on the very long boat ride over. Now that's dedication!

Unfortunately, the majority of wheat grown in the United States contains GMOs (genetically modified organisms) and is heavily doused with the toxic *glyphosate*. Gluten intolerance and sensitivity has been linked to glyphosate consumption, and many gluten intolerant or sensitive people experience great improvement when they stop consuming bread—even sourdough. Other people who are not gluten sensitive actually just experience the ill effects of these chemicals and feel better when they eat organic wheat. However, in my three decades of working with nutrition, I've seen marked improvements in the health of almost everyone who I've encouraged to stop eating gluten, as it's difficult for the body to process and can cause gas, bloating, irritable bowel syndrome, brain fog, lethargy and a host of other symptoms. Because of these factors, the benefits of sourdough simply don't outweigh the downsides of gluten consumption, and you're better off sticking to your own pickled vegetables, plant-based yogurts and of course, kimchi! I don't recommend eating sourdough or any other product made with wheat unless you're quite certain that you don't have any issues from consuming it.

Sauerkraut

Another fermented food that you're probably familiar with is sauerkraut, the fermented cabbage dish that's believed to have originated in Germany. Similar to Kimchi, it's made by fermenting shredded cabbage in a salt water brine (made with table salt or sea salt and water) for a few days or weeks. It's very easy to make at home, tastes tangy and a bit sweet, and starts out with a nice crunch. As time goes on, the cabbage will become softer and softer. Many people enjoy it on sandwiches or as a side dish. Today you can find sauerkraut in just about any grocery store, but once again, much of it has been pasteurized, eliminating many of its nutrients and all of its probiotics. The lesson is simple: homemade is best. Always opt for raw, unpasteurized fermented vegetables (preferably organic) for the most health benefits. Sauerkraut is probably the best fermented food next to kimchi because of its nutritional profile and the other ingredients that go into it.

Kefir & Kvass

Two heavily consumed non-alcoholic fermented beverages are milk kefir and kvass, which both hail from Russia originally. Kefir is a fermented dairy beverage made with cow's, goat's, or sheep's milk. Once fermented for a few days at room temperature, it thickens from its original state, but is usually still drinkable and pourable. Kvass was traditionally made from rye or other naturally leavened bread fermented in water, but more recently it's also being made with beets and other fruits and vegetables. If you want to have kefir, try for the plant-based versions. Homemade kvass with beets can also be delicious—just be sure not to use bread if you're gluten-sensitive.

Kombucha

While kombucha might seem like a healthy option, I've seen numerous patients who drink it regularly experience excess yeast and bacterial overgrowth in their gut. This has been confirmed by lab stool tests through my clinical practice. The excess of yeast and bacteria can lead to SIBO (small intestine bacterial overgrowth) and SIFO (small intestine fungal overgrowth) that throws off the entire microbiome out of balance. Kombucha also has alcohol and often lots of sugar. I therefore recommend avoiding kombucha.

These are just a few examples of fermented foods and beverages which have been staples in the human diet around the world for thousands of years, and hopefully will continue to for many thousands to come.

Kimchi: One Superfood to Rule Them All

So what makes kimchi unique in a world of dozens of other fermented foods? Why is it a superfood not only on par with, but even better for you than yogurt, sourdough, kefir and sauerkraut?

The first thing to note is that kimchi blends several ingredients together, so you're getting all the vitamins and nutrients of everything added to the mix. Whereas sauerkraut

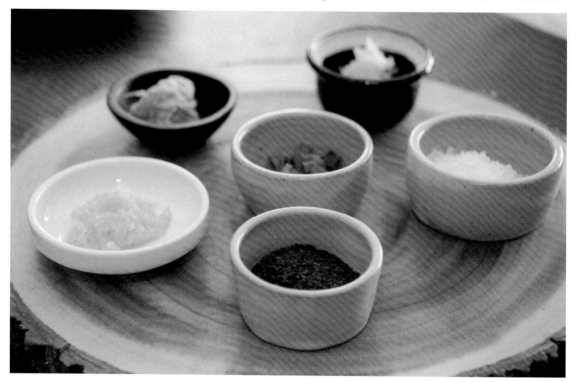

When you eat the traditional bae-chu-kimchi, you not only get the benefits of the napa cabbage, but also of the radishes, green onions, garlic, ginger, red pepper powder, seafood and other ingredients in there.

gives you the health benefits of cabbage, kimchi is the result of teamwork. When you eat the traditional *baechu-kimchi*, you not only get the benefits of the napa cabbage, but also of the radishes, green onions, garlic, ginger, red pepper powder, seafood and other ingredients in there. Let's break it down a bit and explore the health benefits of each ingredient separately.

We'll look at the most familiar of all kimchis, *baechu-kimchi*. The napa cabbage has vitamin C and carotene, which the body converts to vitamin A. Radishes also have lots of vitamin C and minerals like calcium and phosphorous, which helps build bones. Red peppers have many vitamins and are one of the main reasons that harmful bacteria don't grow in kimchi, while helpful bacteria do. *Jeotgal*, fermented seafood, adds flavor and essential amino acids, which can boost the immune system, build muscle and more. However, it's not essential and kimchi can be made 100% vegan. Garlic is one of the world's best anti-microbial foods with high amounts of allicin, which "binds to harmful substances in the human body and allows them to be discharged, thereby detoxifying the body of heavy metals and other such harmful substances."[4] Spring onions contain allicin as well, and like garlic can help ward off harmful bacteria growing in the fermented mix. As you can see, no other fermented food in the world which relies only on single ingredients can compete with this blend of vitamins, minerals, and amino acids. Don't forget that you can also substitute pumpkins, persimmons, or a whole host of other vegetables for napa cabbage, and enjoy the particular health benefits of those foods throughout the year as well.

The second benefit of kimchi is that it's low-calorie, all-natural and mostly plant-based, which also makes it more filling. Before the rise of industrialization during the sixties and seventies, Koreans didn't suffer from nearly the same degree of modern epidemics like heart disease, obesity, and high blood pressure as they do now. Even now, their numbers are comparatively low compared to Americans. Remember, most Koreans traditionally ate some type of kimchi at nearly every meal and this practice continues to this day. Some estimates say that the *average* daily consumption of kimchi has gone from around 300 grams to 60-100 grams nowadays.[5] That means that traditionally Koreans would eat vegetables throughout the day, and that they'd fill themselves up on fiber-rich kimchi loaded with *billions* of probiotic organisms, rather than eating potentially unhealthy foods like the burgers, pizza, bagels and pasta, which are so prevalent in the standard American diet. The average serving (one cup) of kimchi has between 45–90 calories. If we take the low figure, 45 calories, that's about the same as four potato chips. Imagine how quickly you can fill up on a serving of kimchi versus eating only four chips! Even one cup of yogurt has 100 calories and would probably not fill you up nearly as much as a serving of kimchi. It should be no wonder that by eating lots of

Over 2,300 strains of lactic acid bacteria have been found in kimchi!

cabbage, radish and other vegetables, Koreans were able to fill up with great foods while keeping their weight low.

The third benefit of kimchi is similar to that of the other fermented foods: the lactic acid bacteria and other probiotics produced in the fermentation process. Probiotics have been linked to a bunch of health benefits, which will be discussed in Chapter 2. But briefly, our intestinal tract is filled with trillions of bacteria—many of them helpful and some harmful. These bacteria help with everything from digestion to energy production to mood regulation, via the vagus nerve that connects to the brain. The more bad bacteria, pathogenic yeasts, parasites and viruses overgrow in our gut, the more things that can go wrong with our health. Bloating, digestive issues, inflammation and even anxiety and depression can result from microbial imbalances. By eating kimchi, we consume thousands of different strains of beneficial bacteria. In fact, over 2,300 strains of lactic acid bacteria have been found in kimchi! Compare this to the five or so strains that most probiotic pills give you. You just can't compete with real, fermented foods. Plus, you get all of the benefits from eating real, whole, raw and living foods.

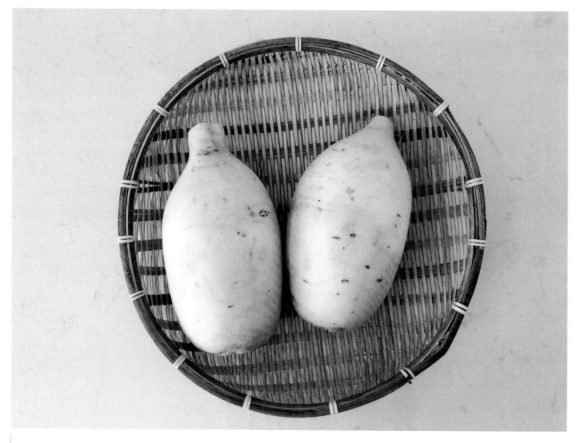

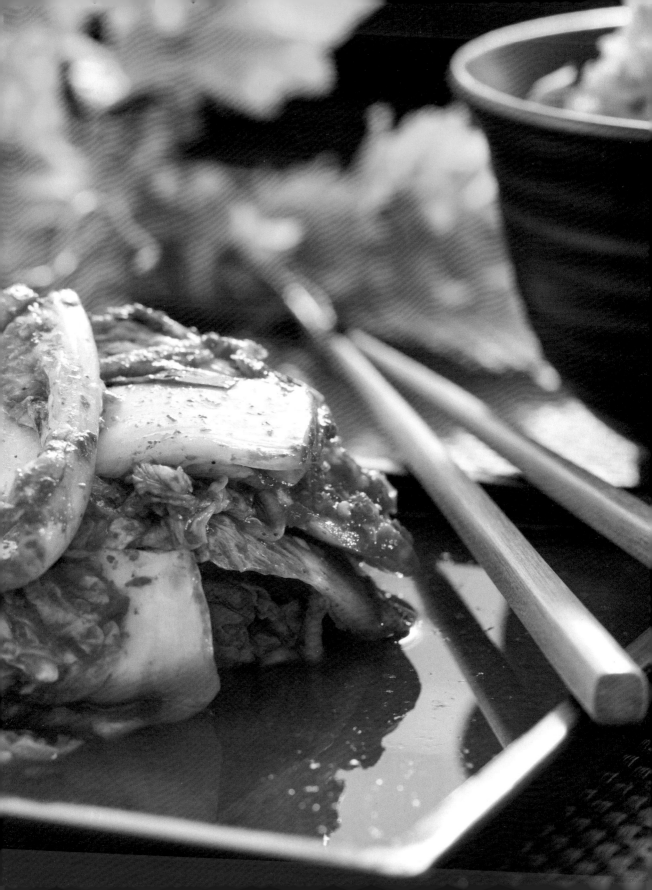

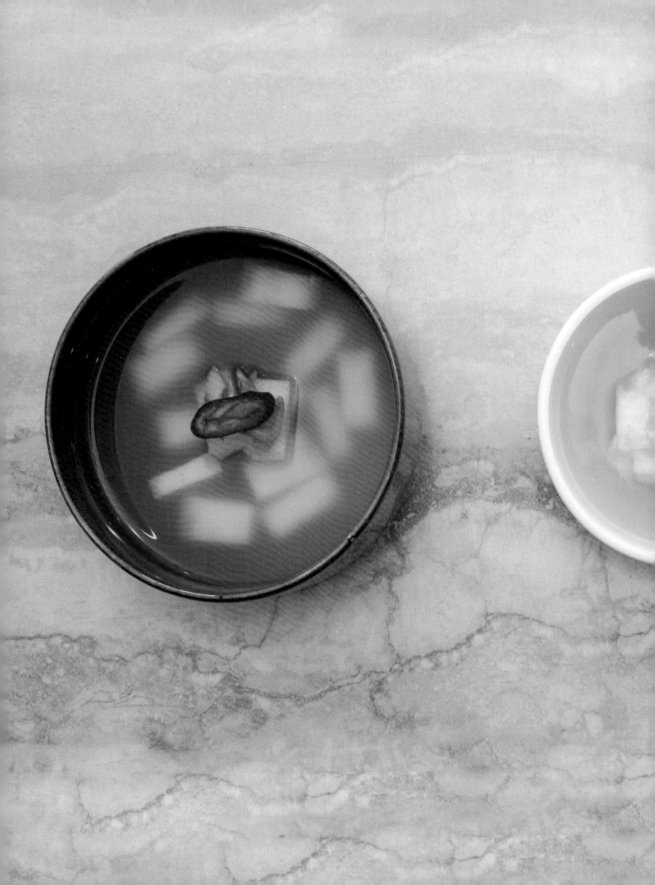

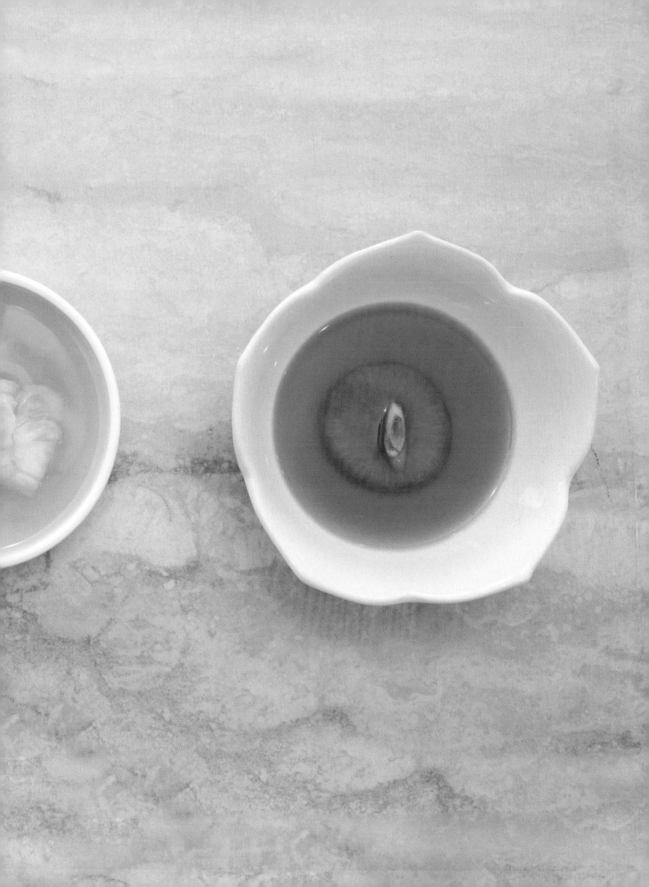

Chapter 2

Kimchi Science & Health Benefits

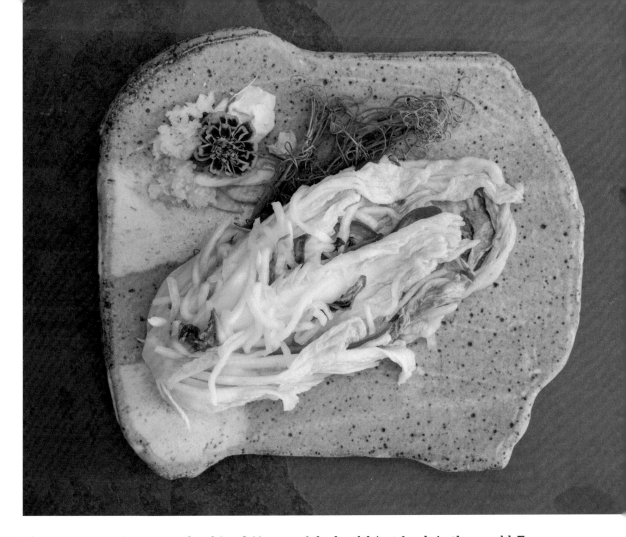

It's no exaggeration to say that kimchi is one of the healthiest foods in the world. Everyone knows that vegetables are super healthy on their own, especially leafy greens like napa cabbage, which makes up the majority of kimchi recipes. But once transformed by lactic acid bacteria through the miraculous process of fermentation, humble veggies become something even greater, something capable of improving and maintaining our health more than the vegetables in their original state.

Kimchi is naturally cholesterol-free (if made vegan), low in fat and calories and packed full of fiber and a wide array of vitamins, minerals and phytochemicals. It also has all the nutritional advantages of ginger, garlic, red peppers, scallions and whatever other vegetables you choose—all wrapped into one. We'll discuss some of these benefits of these other ingredients below.

Here's the nutritional breakdown of a ½ cup of napa cabbage (baechu) kimchi according to SELF Nutrition Data:[1]

Nutrient	Amount	Daily Value
Calories	95.6	5%
Carbohydrates	19.7g	7%
Fiber	2.4g	10%
Protein	3.2g	6%
Total Fat	1.2g	2%
Iron	2.1mg	12%
Manganese	0.5mg	25%
Copper	0.2mg	8%
Calcium	62.8mg	6%
Magnesium	35.0mg	9%
Phosphorus	56.7mg	6%
Potassium	238mg	7%
Sodium	2206mg	92%
Selenium	3.9mcg	6%
Zinc	0.5mg	4%
Folate	83.3mcg	21%
Vitamin B3	1.7mg	9%
Vitamin B5	0.3mg	3%
Vitamin B2	0.1mg	5%
Vitamin B1	0.1mg	9%
Vitamin A	2273IU	45%
Vitamin B6	0.3mg	13%
Vitamin C	12.3mg	21%
Vitamin E	1.4mg	7%
Vitamin K	21.1mcg	26%
Choline	5.6mg	N/A
Betaine	0.1mg	N/A

As you can see, you can get almost half of your vitamin A needs met from a ½ cup of kimchi, 21% of your vitamin C, and a whole range of B vitamins and minerals like potassium, phosphorus and magnesium—all for 96 little calories! Just think of how small a ½ cup is—about eight tablespoons. Generally, I start people off eating only one to two tablespoons a day until they adapt to the fermentation, easing them in to the process of transforming their gut biome. But even at that level, kimchi is truly a wonder food. The more you eat, the better for your body. But the vitamins and minerals are only part of the story. One of the best parts of kimchi comes from its probiotics—the helpful bacteria that scientists are just now linking to a whole host of biological functions, including improved immunity, lower inflammation, better mood and improved digestion.

The Miraculous Human Microbiome

By now, most people in the United States have probably heard about probiotics and how important it is to have healthy gut bacteria. Our gut microbiome consists of the universe of microorganisms that live in each of our bodies, mostly in our large intestine. The collection of these microorganisms numbers over 100 trillion and can weigh up to five pounds! A shocking statistic that made the rounds online was that we have ten times as many bacterial cells in our bodies as we do human cells, but more recent studies suggest that it may actually be closer to a 1:1 ratio between human and bacterial cells in our bodies. Regardless, that means we're just as much "bacteria" as we are "human." So doesn't it make sense to do everything in our power to help foster beneficial bacteria and eliminate harmful ones? Once again, the power of kimchi is up to the task!

Our gut microbiome consists of the universe of microorganisms that live in each of our bodies, mostly in our large intestine. The collection of these microorganisms numbers over 100 trillion and can weigh up to five pounds!

Yet, studying the gut microbiome is still one of the most cutting-edge sectors of scientific research, and scientists have only just begun to uncover all of the roles that these bacteria play in our biological processes. Although the study of the human microbiome began at least several hundred years ago by one of the first microbiologists in the world, Antonie van Leeuwenhoek, it was sidelined as scientists instead focused on the organ systems, brain function and macrological aspects of the human body. The Dutch scientist van Leeuwenhoek, now known as "The Father of Microbiology", was mesmerized by the bacteria in the human body, as he was one of the first people to ever see them. He said of these microbes: "I then most always saw, with great wonder, that in the said matter there were many very little living animalcules, very prettily a-moving."

We've learned a lot since van Leeuwenhoek's time, and in the last few decades especially, scientists all over the world are spending their careers studying the human microbiome. They're busy sequencing an almost infinite number of bacterial, viral, fungi, and protozoa strains that inhabit our bodies. They're also trying to understand what role each of these microorganisms plays in our health and our bodily functions. So far, there are very strong indications that our microbiome is critical to our health and that the bacteria and other species that call our gut home are actually doing a lot to help us.

Our mitochondria—the powerhouses of our cells—are ancient prokaryotes. These evolved microbes symbiotically joined forces with pretty much every cell of our body to provide us with energy and in return would receive protection from the outer elements. They now make up about 10% of our total bodily mass. Just think how important microbes are to our survival!

So what do gut bacteria actually do? We're really just beginning to understand their many functions, but it's clear that when we have too many of the wrong types of bacteria in our gut, or not enough of the good ones, chaos ensues in the form of everything from weight issues to digestive problems to allergies. We also know that good gut bacteria do a lot of positive things for our body, including fighting bad bacteria, processing sugars, lowering inflammation and improving our immune system.

Harvard Medical School cites a study showing that there is "some evidence that a particular strain of the bacterium *Lactobacillus johnsonii* may protect against some cancers," and another study revealed that the bacteria strain "*Akkermansia muciniphila* could prevent inflammation that contributes to fatty plaque buildup in arteries," which is a leading cause of heart disease.[2] Other studies have shown how an overabundance of pathogenic gut bacteria may be linked to "chronic diseases, such as inflammatory bowel disease, obesity, cancer and autism."[3] Studies such as these have cast the role of probiotics—bacteria beneficial to human function—into the limelight. Food manufacturers are eager to advertise their probiotic content in kombucha, yogurt and sauerkraut, and people spend *billions* of dollars annually on probiotic supplements. As I've mentioned, I don't recommend drinking kombucha in particular, due to the potential for yeast and bacterial overgrowth, as well as its high sugar and alcohol content.

You can get the same amount of probiotic bacteria in just one jar of kimchi or sauerkraut as you could get in eight to ten bottles of probiotic supplements!

Early adopters have been taking probiotic supplements in capsule form for a decade or more. What they may not realize though, is that it's much less expensive and more effective to eat raw, fermented foods than to take probiotic supplements. You can get the same amount of probiotic bacteria in just one jar of kimchi or sauerkraut as you could get in eight to ten bottles of probiotic supplements! And the ingredients to make that one jar of kimchi or sauerkraut don't cost more than a few dollars at most.

Study after study has shown that one of the fastest and most effective ways to change our gut biome is to change what we eat. Babies who are fed breast milk versus traditional formulas develop different quantities of the predominant gut bacteria and "the short-term consumption of diets composed entirely of animal meat, eggs, and cheeses or plant-rich in grains, legumes, fruits, and vegetables, altered microbial community structure and overwhelmed inter-individual differences in microbial gene expression."[4] That means that more important than any inborn bacterial differences in individuals were the effects of their diets—whether plant-based or protein-based. This is not to say that we shouldn't eat healthful meats like fish or free-range beef. What it does mean is that integrating more plant foods and fermented foods like kimchi can make a huge difference in changing our internal biome. What you'll learn in this book can change your gut biome in days and weeks (not years), so you can feel the beneficial effects of kimchi that Koreans have known about for centuries.

Kimchi: Why Ingredients Matter

Organic foods have been shown to have many health benefits over the years, but science still needs further testing in order to establish the full range of advantages organic food has over conventionally grown products. However, many health benefits have been firmly established. Some chemicals, such as glyphosate, the world's most commonly used herbicide, are considered "probable carcinogens" by the World Health Organization and this chemical is often sprayed all over conventionally grown wheat fields and more. Roundup® in particular has come under increased scrutiny for its harmful effects.[5] This alone is a good reason to buy organic produce whenever possible.

Conventionally grown vegetables may also not be as nutritious for us as their organic counterparts. A six-year study of onions showed 20% more antioxidants in organic onions versus conventionally grown.[6] Remember, antioxidants are responsible for attacking "free radicals," unstable molecules that bond quickly to areas in the body and produce cellular degeneration. Free radicals are caused by things like radiation, cigarette smoke, drugs and pesticides. These free radicals cause oxidative stress, leading to a "rusting" effect in the body, which can play a role in a host of diseases, such as:

A six-year study of onions showed 20% more antioxidants in organic onions versus conventionally grown.

- Alzheimer's
- Arthritis
- Cancer
- Heart Disease
- Lupus[7]

Free radicals are also known to have an impact on premature aging, as they wear down the body over time if they're not "captured" and dealt with by antioxidants. With organic foods, including the organic vegetables in kimchi, you may be getting more antioxidants, which are one of their main health benefits. By avoiding pesticides, you're also cutting down on your exposure to free radicals.

So it's especially important to use organic ingredients for all the kimchi you make. While many people are beginning to understand the health benefits of organic foods in general, new research has been done looking into its effects on kimchi and probiotic production in particular. A study entitled "Physiochemical and Quality Characteristics of Young Radish (Yulmoo) Kimchi Cultivated by Organic Farming" (2014) shows how organic radishes outperformed control groups of conventionally grown radishes in terms of producing more helpful bacteria and increasing the freshness of kimchi and its nutritional content.[8] Perhaps unsurprisingly, helpful bacteria find it easier to grow on food that has not been sprayed with pesticides and chemicals, whose aim is to kill or deter various life forms. Not only that, but participants in the study found the organic kimchi to be more aesthetically pleasing as well! By using organic cabbage, radishes, peppers and other ingredients, you can maximize the health potential of your kimchi and make it easier on the body, since it won't have to use valuable resources to deal with pesticides and toxicants.

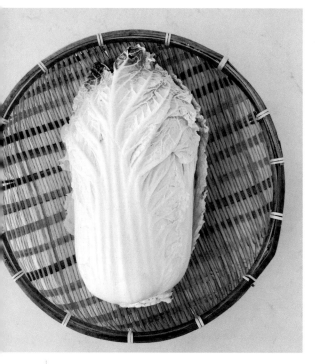

Washing, seasoning and brining have been shown to decrease up to 85% of pesticide traces on cabbage and radishes in the preparation of kimchi.

There's good news, however. Even if you use conventional vegetables or some pesticides have "drifted" onto the vegetables you use, the process of preparing kimchi can actually reduce the amount of leftover residue. Washing, seasoning and brining have been shown to decrease up to 85% of pesticide traces on cabbage and radishes in the preparation of kimchi.[9] Lactic acid bacteria go on to break down much of the remaining portion. Using organic ingredients helps the environment, but it helps your internal environment too.

Which type of salt you choose is also important. While it might not seem like a big deal, choosing the wrong salt can affect the taste, look and overall outcome of your kimchi. A study done in Korea tested different salt types for both acidity levels and how people reacted to each one after a taste test.[10] Purified salt, the type most readily available in supermarkets and at restaurants, was contrasted with sea salt for the purposes of the study. What the researches found was that using purified salt spiked acid levels more quickly and also made the kimchi soggier more quickly. By

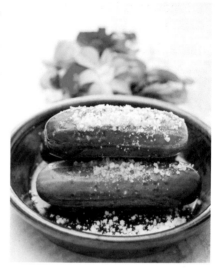

contrast, sea salt helped keep the kimchi crisper and acid levels rose only gradually. Refined table salt, if it's iodized, can also be a problem. Once again, participants preferred the kimchi made with sea salt over the one made with purified salt.[11] But not all sea salts are the same. Himalayan salt has around 95% sodium chloride, with low levels of minerals, while other salts can be only 70% sodium chloride with higher amounts of calcium, magnesium and phosphorus. Solar sea salt—and Korean or Celtic solar sea salt in particular—is best.

Kimchi's Fermentation Process

So how does kimchi undergo fermentation and what exactly does this magical process do to the healthful properties of the cabbages, radishes, garlic, ginger and/or peppers that you bite into weeks after they've been stored? At the most basic level, fermentation is the process whereby bacteria break down the sugars in food in order to feed themselves, and they do so anaerobically—without oxygen. As a result of this process, they emit alcohols, gases or acid in the process. When they emit alcohol, you get beer, wine, spirits or Korea's favorite, *soju*. When we ferment foods, we're encouraging certain types of bacteria to grow. Temperature, pH, oxygen levels and the length of fermentation all play a role in how quickly or slowly these bacteria grow.

Over time, if you've made it right, these bacteria then outnumber and overtake the bacteria that would normally result in the decomposition and putrefaction of food, and along with brining, the bacteria help to preserve the kimchi for longer. The bacteria that grow on kimchi are types of *probiotics*, and in addition to helping our food last longer, these beneficial bacteria are good for our gut, immune system,

You don't need a starter for kimchi—the lactic acid bacteria on your hands and on the vegetables is enough!

digestion and more. Kimchi is host to a variety of types of bacteria, and members of *Leuconostoc*, *Lactobacillus* and *Weissella* genus dominate, each at different times in the fermentation process.[12] And each of these types of bacteria have many health advantages for your body. For instance, lactobacillus may reduce cholesterol, fight off colds and flus, aid in weight loss and reduce allergies and eczema, along with improving overall gut health.[13] One can also use lactic acid bacteria starters to speed the process along, although this is mainly used in commercial kimchi production. You don't need a starter for kimchi—the lactic acid bacteria on your hands and on the vegetables is enough! Just in case you have any skin issues, such as eczema, psoriasis or fungal infections, it's best to use gloves so as not to spoil the fermentation process.

The main complaint of over-fermentation is what it does to the taste. Letting the kimchi ferment too long can produce an increasingly sour or acidic taste, due to the buildup of compounds that the bacteria release. However, improper fermentation methods in commercial production have been linked to E. coli and norovirus outbreaks, although these are *extremely* uncommon, because the probiotics in kimchi do such a good job of attacking and overpowering any harmful bacteria that might grow on the kimchi due to contamination. Still, this is another good reason to make it at home. Kimchi—between its pH and lactic acid bacteria content—is extremely safe, killing off most harmful bacteria and organisms.

Health Benefits of Kimchi

There are almost infinite potential health benefits that can come from eating kimchi on a regular basis. Most of these benefits have studies to back them up as I discuss below. Other benefits, not discussed here since they've not been scientifically verified, have been passed down as sacred knowledge throughout many generations in Korea and beyond. Everyday, scientists are verifying more and more of what Koreans innately know about how good kimchi is, and I wouldn't be surprised to see an increasing amount of the literature validate this folk wisdom as the years go on.

These are just some of the many benefits—backed by scientific studies—that you can look forward to after making kimchi a regular part of your diet:

- Gut Health and Stronger Immunity
- Enhanced Digestion and Elimination
- Weight Loss and Body Contouring

- Cardiovascular Health
- Anti-Aging and Antioxidant Properties
- Greater Energy
- Clearer, Vibrant Skin
- Mood Enhancer
- Increased Mental Clarity
- Healthy Blood Pressure
- Anti-Mutagenic and Cancer Prevention

Now let's take a closer look at each of these life-changing benefits in order to understand kimchi's power to transform your health.

Gut Health, Immunity and SIBO

Eating kimchi is one of the best things you can do to help your immune system. Besides being rich in vitamin C, kimchi is also host to probiotics like lactic acid bacteria, the same ones found in yogurt. Put simply, when these good bacteria outnumber and dominate harmful bacteria, yeasts and parasites—including the kind that make us sick or hurt our immune functioning—we feel better.

What most people don't know is that about 70-80% of our immune system is actually located in our gut. This is known as the Gut Associated Lymphoid Tissue (GALT). It's where the struggle between probiotics and harmful bacteria and viruses—the ones that cause colds and flus—most often play out. Our gut is often referred to as our second brain, and for good reason—our gut is seriously smart when it comes to fighting disease! Many of our neurotransmitters and immune fighting compounds like antibodies are produced by cells in our small intestines, the longest organ in our body.[14] The power of billions of live probiotic bacteria present in each serving of kimchi, along with an astounding array of vitamins, minerals and countless phytonutrients makes for a serious contender against any unruly virus, bacteria or fungi that may try to wreak havoc in your body. A study found that one of the prominent species of lactic acid bacteria in kimchi, called L. *Mesenteroides*, produces cyclic dipeptides which exhibit antimicrobial activity (Liu et al. 2017).[15] And a stronger immune system, with less microbes attacking it, is much better equipped to prevent any sort of serious health issues like cancer, as we'll talk more about later.

Our gut biome and the types of bacteria we inherit is passed onto us by our mothers from birth. Therefore, the relative health of your mother's gut bacteria can determine yours at an early age.

Our gut microbiome is also responsible for many important functions related to healthy immunity. Our gut biome and the types of bacteria we inherit is passed onto us by our mothers from birth. Therefore, the relative health of your mother's gut bacteria can determine yours at an early age. Likewise, for female readers, what you eat now can help strengthen the microbiome of any children you may plan on having in the future. As Broussard and Devkota have shown, a whole list of modern epidemics, from Diabetes to irritable bowel syndrome (IBS) to allergies and more may be traceable to the difference between the types of bacteria humans traditionally had and the new types of gut biomes that arose due to industrialized food production and modern lifestyles.[16] In other words, we've altered our gut biomes throughout history and inherited new bacteria from our mothers—not all of which are ideal for helping to process foods and fight against disease. In particular, the authors show how easier access to refined sugars and simple carbohydrates has become a dominant feature of the Western diet and how the move away from fiber-rich foods allows unhealthy gut biomes to flourish. The scientists remark that:

> Additional insights, however, can be gained from the human studies looking at metabolic disease incidence in Western versus non-Western dietary traditions. A unifying theme among these native populations, irrespective of geographic location, is that diabetes and obesity is nearly unheard of (pg. 739).[17]

Again, the prevalence of bacteria closer to those of our original ancestors' diets—focused on local, organic, fiber-rich, unprocessed foods—seems to help people thrive. The healthier the gut bacteria and diversity, the less likelihood of diabetes and obesity, so it seems. In terms of its ability to be made naturally, its probiotic content, *and* its fiber, kimchi is a clear winner!

But there's more. In some people, an excess consumption of carbohydrates and sugars can lead to an overgrowth of bacteria in the small intestine, known as SIBO (small intestinal bacterial overgrowth), as the bacteria feed off of sugars. SIBO has only recently come to be understood as a more common diagnosis—the result of excess bacteria taking over. It's been linked by Dukowicz, Lacy and Levine (2014) to irritable bowel syndrome, as well as "frequently implicated as the cause of chronic diarrhea and malabsorption. Patients with SIBO may also suffer from unintentional weight loss, nutritional deficiencies and osteoporosis" (pg. 112).[18] However, SIBO has been correlated with a bunch of more serious conditions. One study found that there's a strong correlation between restless leg syndrome and SIBO, as well as irritable bowel syndrome.[19] In a 2015 study, a quarter of patients with unexplained GI symptoms like bloating, gas and nausea were found to have SIFO (Small Intestinal Fungal Overgrowth), also known as Candidiasis.[20] But the effects of SIBO go even deeper. A significant number (44%) of Type 1 Diabetics who suffer from autonomic neuropathy were found to also have SIBO. The study found that those patients had a higher daily insulin requirement than Type 1 Diabetics without autonomic neuropathy.[21] If this sounds like you, kimchi can be helpful when introduced into your diet, along with a corresponding decrease in your sugar intake. The less sugar you eat, the less harmful fungi and bacteria grow. And the more probiotic-rich foods like kimchi you eat, the more the lactic acid bacteria can help fight the bad guys off.

Finally, a 2016 study of Chinese patients with MS (Multiple Sclerosis) found that 38% tested positive for SIBO, compared to 8% in the control group.[22] Again, the casual relationship is not clear, but there seems to be a connection between bacterial overgrowth and a host of health issues. Further study is needed in order to determine the exact connection, but the good news is that kimchi can help to relieve both problems.

There's yet another reason why kimchi is so essential for our gut health, especially in terms of boosting our immunity. We've reached a point in our medical system where antibiotics have lost much of their effectiveness due to overuse, resulting in the development of "superbugs", pathogenic bacteria which are now incredibly resistant to antibiotics as they mutate over time. Instead of being easily treated with antibiotics, these superbugs are able to progress and grow unchecked. Unfortunately, this means that people are dying from infections that not long ago were easily cured with a prescription for an antibiotic. Each year in the United States alone, more than two million people become infected with antibiotic-resistant bacteria, and more than 23,000 of them die from these infections.[23]

With this huge health threat looming, it's more important than ever to strengthen your immune system naturally with wholesome foods, daily exercise, plenty of quality sleep and stress reduction. Then, when you're exposed to a potentially life-threatening bacteria, your immune system will be better able to defend itself from the invader. You'll be happy to know that kimchi is also believed to boost white blood cell and immune cell development—meaning more cells to fight off harmful bacteria and viruses.[24]

It's more important than ever to strengthen your immune system naturally with wholesome foods, daily exercise, plenty of quality sleep and stress reduction.

I recommend daily kimchi consumption for this purpose, as it's one of the very best immune system boosters that I've found in all my years of practice, and it's so simple and inexpensive to incorporate into your life—not to mention mouth-wateringly delicious.

"Will The Diarrhea Ever Stop?"

Teddy, a forty-six year old male CEO was suffering from a serious case of diarrhea. He would go to the bathroom 10–12 times a day and dealt with everything from loose stools to watery, projectile diarrhea. His symptoms started six months prior to seeing me, after three rounds of antibiotics for a chronic sinus infection. The same doctor who prescribed him the antibiotics told him he might be suffering from an irritable bowel due to his stressful job, so he recommended that Teddy take an over the counter pink liquid to stop the diarrhea. He presented to my office frustrated and exhausted from his condition and wanted to get to the root cause of his diarrhea.

I run a stool analysis for all of my patients with diarrhea, looking for pathogenic bacteria and parasites, and sure enough the results were positive for a *Clostridium difficile* (C. diff) infection. I explained to him that this microbe naturally lives in the human intestinal tract, but can become a pathogenic infection—one of the side effects of oral antibiotics. I also told him that he had a choice to go back to the internist for more drugs or try my natural healing approach. He had no interest in getting another antibiotic.

I had treated many individuals with C. diff. before and gotten excellent results, so I was excited to help him feel better quickly. The first step was to clean up his diet, so I had him eliminate any inflammatory foods that were irritating his gut and feeding the C. diff bacteria. This is the same anti-inflammatory diet that I recommend in Chapter 3 of this book. I also recommended a natural herbal formula that would mitigate the C. diff infection without irritating his already inflamed gut.

Second, we needed to re-inoculate his digestive system with lactic acid bacteria to help control the C. diff. infection quickly. He tried taking probiotics in the past, but they didn't make much of an impact. I mentioned that he needed much higher levels than what's typically found in supplements, and the best way to get high levels of probiotics is by following The Kimchi Diet™. He was reluctant to make his own kimchi, but I told him that if he followed my kimchi recipe and consumed it as directed, he would start feeling better again. And that's all he wanted: to have normal bowel movements again!

I saw him exactly ten days later, and I could tell from his face that he was really excited to see me. His watery diarrhea had stopped after eating kimchi for five days straight. The consistency was more like "mud" and his bowel movements went down to only three times a day. Plus, the sinus symptoms completely cleared up without any medication. This was a huge improvement to him, considering all that he went through for months.

We continued on The Kimchi Diet™ for another two months and not only did his C.diff. infection clear up completely during the second month (which was confirmed by another stool test), he also believes that kimchi saved his life. He still eats kimchi every day!

Reduced Inflammation

Inflammation is one of the root causes of so many conditions that afflict us. As I trace out in *The 7-Day Allergy Makeover*, when our body comes into contact with substances that it can't process easily, it often produces an inflammatory response. It's your body's way of trying to fight off these chemicals or toxicants—just like when you get sick. Eat enough processed food or food that you're sensitive to (gluten, dairy, sugar, soy, etc.), live in a place surrounded by dust mites, pet dander or environmental pollutants and that inflammatory response can make you start to feel sick and sluggish. It saps your body of its vital resources to fight *real* diseases when they do come along. It's why I've seen so many people with allergies get sick every couple of months—because their bodies are using all their energy to fight off the allergies when they should be fighting disease. Not only that, Kim et al. (2014) have found a correlation between kimchi consumption and asthma incidence. Essentially, the more kimchi you eat, the less your chance of suffering from asthma.[25] The same is true of rhinitis, according to a 2016 study.[26] Fortunately, for those suffering from allergies, Rho et. al (2017) have shown that a specific microbe found in kimchi called *Enterococcus faecium* FC-K has anti-allergenic effects by reducing levels of IgE (Immunoglobulin E) in the body.[27] IgE is an important marker for inflammation and allergies, so lower levels are a good thing.

Inflammation can also lead to joint and muscle pain, swelling and a host of other discomforts. Chronic inflammation has been linked to arthritis, many autoimmune disorders and even some forms of cancer. It's why in Chapter 3 you'll read about my *Anti-Inflammatory Diet*, a variation of what I recommend all my patients adopt, since it nourishes your body with only the healthiest foods and cuts out as many possible irritants and allergens as possible. It's also the diet that I used to heal my son Cody's allergies, and it's helped thousands of my patients suffering not only from allergies, but from other inflammatory issues like arthritis, fibromyalgia and autoimmune disorders.

Of course, kimchi is a big part of my Anti-Inflammatory Diet. And the science backs it up. Not only does kimchi contain garlic and ginger, which are two of the single best anti-inflammatory foods you can eat, but cabbage in particular is a lesser known anti-inflammatory and antioxidant food. There are also anti-inflammatory chemicals found in kimchi that help to protect against oxidative stress (which causes aging and many forms of disease) in the body.[28] But kimchi itself has been shown to help with inflammation because of its probiotic content. Studies have shown that many times, inflammatory responses are linked to a microbial imbalance in the gut,[29] and increasing probiotic intake is one of the most promising new areas of scientific research for treating inflammation.[30] All this means that restoring your good gut bacteria through kimchi may be one of the best things you can do for your inflammation.

Kimchi may be one of the best things you can do for your inflammation.

Autoimmune or Just Inflamed?

Susan was a 36 year old mother of 6 year old twin boys and complained of sleep deprivation, constipation and muscle aches all over her body. She thought her stiffness and pain was from lack of exercise and the extra fifteen pounds of weight she'd not been able to shed since her pregnancy. She stated that she had a poor diet of sugar and snacks and didn't move around much—except when she was chasing after her boys!

Her physical exam was unremarkable except that her abdomen was bloated around her waistline. When I measured her waist and hip circumference, it was 36 inches in the waist and 34 inches in the hips. This indicated that her abdomen was either distended from an inflamed gut or from excess fat accumulation. Either way, she was not happy with her body and wanted to feel better.

I ordered all appropriate blood tests to rule out any issues including thyroid disease, anemia, blood sugar imbalances, autoimmune issues and more.

The only biomarker that was positive was the ANA, antinuclear antibodies test, which indicated that she was experiencing some form of autoimmune attack on her own tissues, hence the pain all over her body. I followed up with another blood test to find out what specific type of autoimmune disease it might point toward: rheumatoid arthritis, lupus, Sjogren's disease and so on. But all tests were negative, which was actually a good thing.

I suspected that she had gut issues and suffered from systemic inflammation from the poor eating habits. Lifestyle changes were in order.

I put her on The Kimchi Diet™, with some digestive supplements, and three weeks into our treatment protocol, Susan's muscle pains had reduced by 75% and her constipation was completely gone. She confessed that she hadn't been this regular since she was in college! She also mentioned that she urinated excessively during the first two weeks, and that she lost a total of seven pounds in that short time. Unbelievable!

After eight weeks of The Kimchi Diet™, she came back into the office and wanted another blood test. Susan was anxious to see if the ANA had changed, since she had been completely free of pain for weeks and was sleeping like a baby. Not only that, her belly was flatter and she had healthy bowel movements daily like clockwork. She had a lot more energy, was happier and ready to start a workout program at the local gym. I wasn't sure if the blood test would change so quickly, but I was pleasantly surprised that she passed her ANA blood test with flying colors!

Anti-Aging and Antioxidant Properties

As discussed, antioxidants are powerful compounds that help your body to fight oxidation or "rust" in the body by capturing free radicals. Free radicals are oxygen-containing molecules that bond easily with other chemicals in the body, setting off harmful chemical reactions and causing cellular damage. Just imagine your body trying going about its normal, healthy functions while it's bombarded with chemicals that can disrupt that functioning and cause degeneration. Now, keep in mind that even eating and breathing naturally cause *some* cellular damage over time, but we greatly speed this process up if we eat bad foods or are exposed to harmful toxicants and pollutants. Aging, at a simple level, is exactly this process of cellular damage caused by free radicals. Some have even suspected that if we could halt the work of free radicals in the body, we'd greatly slow the process of aging. It's why a fifty year old can be "younger" than a thirty-five year old at the biological level: the healthy fifty year old has done less damage to their body in the form of free radical exposure and/or has consumed more foods with antioxidant properties.

Free radical exposure comes in the form of:

- Pollution: Air and Water
- Heavy Metals and Chemicals
- Mold Toxicity

- Over the Counter and Prescription Drugs
- Smoking
- Alcohol
- Many Processed Meats
- Rancid Oils (Olive, Walnut, Avocado, Sesame and Coconut are the best)
- Lifestyle: Not Sleeping Enough, Exercising Too Much

Therefore, to reverse free radical impact and slow the process of aging, we need to minimize our exposure to the above compounds and foods, and we should include antioxidant foods like broccoli, cherries, spinach, blueberries and walnuts in our diet. And by now, you probably won't be surprised to learn that kimchi is one of the best antioxidative foods all around. Park and Ju (2018) show that kimchi has "vitamin C, chlorophyll, phenols, carotenoids, dietary fiber and other phytochemicals", as well as "further metabolites with LAB (lactic acid bacteria)" that have antioxidant and anti-aging properties (pg. 58).[31] This anti-aging quality of kimchi increases as it ripens. Part of Korean folk wisdom is that eating well helps keep you feeling young—and now science has proven it! A new study suggests that kimchi consumption increases compounds like glutathione, the master antioxidant, which is anti-inflammatory and therefore may be helpful in treating and preventing Alzheimer's disease (Woo et al. 2018).[32] It's also been shown to be "neuroprotective" in mice studies, helping in the regeneration of the nervous system.[33]

The high-fiber nature of kimchi also contributes to its anti-aging effects. A high fiber diet has been correlated to an increase in production of butyrate, a short-chain fatty acid (SCFA) produced by the bacterial fermentation of fiber in the colon. The fiber in kimchi feeds the lactic acid bacteria, and the metabolic end product results in an increase of butyrate. Butyrate is a short-chain fatty acid that's related to a decrease in colon disease such as cancer, brain inflammation and more. And butyrate is linked to decreased inflammatory markers in the body.[34] This is important to prevent signs of aging as we get older. Not only that, the benefits of a high-fiber diet for the colon have been well-established, but now there's evidence that a high-fiber diet can positively alter gene expression in the brain, with the potential to treat various neurological disorders that affect us as we get older.[35] You've heard all your life how important fiber is, and now here's your chance to eat lots of it.

A serving of kimchi for all!

Enhanced Digestion and Elimination

I strongly believe that a healthy mind and body begins with optimal digestion, but unfortunately the majority of us lack this essential function. Lots of factors can play into a poor digestive system, such as antibiotic use, excessive stress, lack of quality sleep and eating lots of highly processed food. As they say, all disease begins in the colon.

When we engage in these types of unhealthy activities year after year, our gut microbiome can become seriously imbalanced, with too little of the "good guys" (probiotic bacteria) and too many of the "bad guys" (pathogenic bacteria, fungi, viruses and parasites). When this happens, we can develop so many different ailments, from constipation to bloating and gas to irritable bowel and chronic fatigue syndrome to autoimmune diseases and fibromyalgia. The list of possibilities is almost endless. And because of this, millions of people are suffering needlessly, often for many years.

Often doctors will only prescribe drugs to suppress the symptoms of these diseases, but these quick fix treatments almost never correct the underlying issue, which may be gut dysfunction. In conjunction with making healthier lifestyle choices like getting enough sleep and managing stress effectively, choosing a diet of fresh and fermented whole foods can be of huge benefit in overcoming gut dysfunction and the diseases that often go with it.

Kimchi is a super effective digestive aid, helping to break down carbohydrates and fiber in the grains and veggies that it's often eaten with. The red pepper powder in kimchi helps to stimulate stomach acid production so that we can actually digest our food more effectively. The lactic acid bacteria in kimchi helps to further break down food and to balance our entire gut microbiome as well.[36] It's been shown to lower pH in the colon, which helps to kill harmful organisms there and it also decreases the amount of harmful enzymes.[37] As if that wasn't enough, another study by Marco et al. (2017) found that microorganisms found in fermented foods help to protect against the bowel disease colitis and epithelial cell damage.[38] As of now, we're only aware of a sliver of the benefits that these tiny organisms confer to humans, but we're learning more all the time.

The lactic acid bacteria in kimchi helps to further break down food and to balance our entire gut microbiome.

Salmonellosis Beware!

I'd been taking care of Mark and his family for the past seven years, coming in for various health issues ranging from headaches to allergies to common viral infections.

But this time, I was asked if I could see Mark for an emergency visit. He had a business dinner the night before at a sushi restaurant and woke up in the middle of the night with severe abdominal pain, cramping and diarrhea. The diarrhea wouldn't stop, and he had gone to the bathroom at least seven times before they called me early that morning.

This was most likely a bad case of food poisoning, but I still wanted to send out a stool analysis. Stool tests take time for the results though, and I wanted to help him as quickly as possible. Each time Mark had diarrhea, he was getting weaker and starting to experience headaches and chills.

Salmonella food poisoning is usually a self-limiting condition where the standard of care is to tell the patient to rest, drink a lot of fluids and eat a bland diet. If there isn't any bloody diarrhea or a fever higher than 101.5 degrees Fahrenheit, then the patient is asked to take care of themselves at home.

I recommended that Mark take some oregano oil tablets, a natural antimicrobial agent, for a few days. I also asked Mark's wife, Kerry to pick up some napa cabbage kimchi at the grocery store and buy the one with the most juice in the jar. I had her squeeze out the kimchi juice from the cabbage and feed Mark one tablespoon of the juice every two hours until it was all gone. I told them that he may have one more bout of diarrhea, but afterwards, it would most likely stop. The kimchi juice would calm down his cramps and abdominal pain.

Mark called me the next day thanking me, saying he had followed my recommendation exactly as directed. Sure enough, the kimchi juice did the trick! In fact, he did have one last bout of diarrhea, but felt like it was more of a "purge." His belly felt so relaxed and happy that he went to sleep early and woke up with energy—completely cramp-free and without diarrhea.

Once again, kimchi to the rescue!

Weight Loss, Diabetes and Heart Health

It seems like just about everyone is currently trying to lose excess weight, often to little avail. As of 2014, almost one-third of the global population was overweight or obese, and if we continue on our current path, that number will rise to almost half by 2030.[39] We all know that being overweight or obese is a major contributor to many health problems, including life-threatening diseases like cancer, heart disease, stroke and diabetes. As of 2014 in the United States alone, obesity related medical expenses tallied up to almost

$150 billion![40] And that's just for one year. What a massive unnecessary financial burden is being placed upon us. I bet that those costs have only increased since 2014 and will continue to rise until we get this epidemic under control.

The rise of processed food in the last century has contributed greatly to the obesity epidemic in the United States. This should come as no surprise. A diet consisting of mostly unprocessed, whole foods is the way to go in terms of promoting health and vitality. But what many people don't realize is that fermented foods, which our ancestors ate on a daily basis, are almost totally absent from most people's diets in this country. And I believe that this is another

Kimchi is packed full of fiber, water, vitamins, minerals, phytochemicals, live enzymes and beneficial bacteria, while being very low in fat and calories.

huge contributor to not only to the amount of people dealing with being overweight or obese, but many other health issues as well.

Numerous studies in mice and humans indicate that including kimchi as a regular part of your diet fights obesity and overweight conditions.[41] And it makes sense when you think about it. Kimchi is packed full of fiber, water, vitamins, minerals, phytochemicals, live enzymes and beneficial bacteria, while being very low in fat and calories. Perfect diet food? You bet! When eaten daily, both fresh and fermented kimchi can lower body weight, body mass index and body fat, but the results are much greater with fermented kimchi.[42] Plus, the red pepper powder that's included in many kimchi recipes contains a phytochemical called *capsaicin*, which increases our body's fat burning metabolism. The garlic, radish and ginger also play a role, and perhaps even a larger role in weight loss than red pepper, so even kimchi made without red pepper can help people lose weight.[43] Good news for those

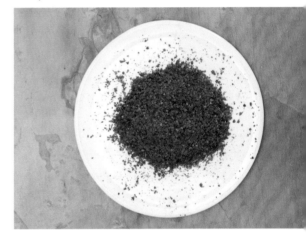

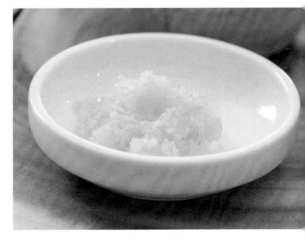

of you who don't like your food too spicy! Suffice to say that kimchi is a total rockstar in the nutrition world and needs to be on everyone's plate.

It's recently been discovered that overweight people have a very different make-up of bacteria in their digestive system than thin people have. But kimchi positively impacts the composition of our gut bacteria, including in people with obesity.[44] Scientists have found that overweight or obese people have lower levels of Bacteroides and higher levels of Firmicutes, but eight weeks of daily kimchi consumption was shown to favorably alter this ratio.[45] And if an overweight person becomes thin, the types and numbers of microorganisms that are found in their gut change dramatically as a result, and vice versa when a thin person becomes overweight.[46] But here's the kicker: they also found that eating kimchi regularly helps to change the gut microbiome to be more in line with that of a thin person's. Jackpot!

Along those lines, many obese people are suffering from diabetes, another disease which is the result of our modern lifestyle and the negative effects it has on our gut bacteria. It's estimated that almost 180 million people globally suffer from diabetes, but many of them are unaware that they even have the condition.[47] High amounts of sugar (also in the form of refined carbohydrates like bread, donuts, pasta, and bagels) not only spike our blood sugar levels, but they feed the bad bacteria in our gut, as discussed above. The body needs more and more sugar to feel normal. In less severe, prediabetic conditions, this might just feel like brain fog or sugar crashes. But in more extreme states, the body becomes unable to regulate its insulin production. Diabetes is the result. The good news is that kimchi—at least those containing napa cabbage—has been shown to help stave off diabetes, even in those who ate a high-fat diet.[48] Fresh and fermented kimchi also can decrease weight, BMI (body mass index), waist circumference, insulin resistance and blood pressure in prediabetic individuals.[49]

For anyone struggling with weight, heart health is a real concern. Kimchi is also excellent for overall heart health, helping by lowering cholesterol and lowering inflammation. Its ability to lower cholesterol levels is one of kimchi's best features for a world overtaken by the obesity crisis. A 2018 study found that certain probiotic microbe strains found in kimchi lowered cholesterol in rats who had hypercholesterolemia (super high cholesterol). The microbes both assimilated excess cholesterol as well as caused the rats to excrete it in their feces.[50] In other words, they could both handle some of the extra cholesterol *and* get rid of some of it in their waste products. An active component of kimchi known as HDMPPA has also shown promise in slowing down the development of fatty streaks in the aortic sinuses of mice fed a high cholesterol containing diet.[51] Another study shows that kimchi, along with lowering cholesterol, also works to lower triglycerides and LDL levels, reducing the risk of heart attack or stroke.[52] Kimchi can be a real life saver by working on some of the harmful compounds in our bodies. Because it lowers cholesterol levels, kimchi also possesses anti-atherosclerotic (heart protective) properties and effects in the body.[53] Heart health begins with kimchi!

Heart health begins with kimchi!

I find it so fascinating to think about the trillions of gut bacteria that we each host in our body and to ponder exactly what they're doing and why. Hopefully time will tell, but we've already started to uncover some of their important functions, and we know for sure that a healthy microbiome is a critical component of our overall health and vitality. Many millions of people struggle year after year trying to lose and keep off excess weight, and unfortunately so many of them are unsuccessful despite their best efforts. Could kimchi and other fermented foods be the missing link to maintaining optimal weight for life? I certainly believe it's an important part of a total lifestyle transformation that shouldn't be underestimated.

Could kimchi and other fermented foods be the missing link to maintaining optimal weight for life?

Energy, Mood and Mental Clarity

Imagine everything that you could accomplish if you had abundant energy each and every day. Or if you could go through it all with a better mood and sense of mental clarity.

I usually zip through my days with vibrant energy, but this is because I've put so much time and effort into my health over the years. But abundant energy wasn't always the norm for me, and it's certainly not the norm for most of the people who come to me for help with their health. We're all overworked and overstressed—and we're paying for it dearly.

However, work and stress aside (though they certainly matter when it comes to how much energy you have), what you choose to eat makes a huge difference in how much energy you have throughout the day. Ideally, you'll want to eat several meals and snacks per day, consisting of unprocessed foods like fresh fruits and vegetables, nuts and seeds, gluten-free whole grains and clean protein, along with a hefty dose of fermented foods like kimchi. These are all discussed in my Anti-Inflammatory Diet in Chapter 3, and I go into more depth on it in *The 7-Day Allergy Makeover*. A combination of these foods will provide your body with a healthy ratio of carbohydrates, protein and fat, as well as the micronutrients your body needs to function optimally for long periods of time.

Over 8% of adults in the United States are suffering from depression, and women are twice as likely as men to be affected by it.[54] If you or anyone you know has dealt with depression, then you know what a challenge it can be. At the other end of the spectrum, anxiety disorders are the most common mental illness in the United States, affecting over 18% of the population each year. And the gut biome is the physiological connection between what we eat and how we feel. As previously mentioned, the vagus nerve, which runs from the gut to the brain, connects our mind to our internal biome, sending messages back and forth. More research shows that the "gastrointestinal tract is sensitive to emotion. Anger, anxiety, sadness, elation—all of these feelings (and others) can trigger symptoms in the gut."[55] Therefore, anxiety can cause reactions in the gut, but likewise, problems in the gut may trigger anxiety or depression. This helps explain why, according to John Hopkins University, a higher percentage of individuals with IBS than a random sample of the population sample develop anxiety or depression.[56]

There's good news, however. Dinan et. al (2013) have come to define a new category of food, *psychobiotics*, which consists of a "live organism that, when ingested in adequate amounts, produces a health benefit in patients suffering from psychiatric illness. As a class of probiotic, these bacteria are capable of producing and delivering neuroactive substances such as gamma-aminobutyric acid (GABA) and serotonin, which act on the brain-gut axis."[57] Since a large variety of antidepressants already work to increase serotonin production (or inhibit its reuptake), Dinan's research opens—or verifies—the connection Koreans have understood between eating kimchi and improved emotional state. But the connection between kimchi and mood goes even further. Specific bacteria present in kimchi have been found to increase GABA production in our brains, also verifying Dinan's research.[58] GABA is a neurotransmitter that's known to induce calmness and relaxation and helps to relieve depression, anxiety, insomnia and more. Lactic acid bacteria isolated from kimchi increase the production of gamma-aminobutyric acid (GABA), which also has a neuroprotective effect on the brain.[59] Getting your gut right with healthy bacteria that come from kimchi will do a lot to enhance your mood and give you that feeling of relaxation and release from pressure we Koreans call *siwonhan-mat*.

Clear Skin

Who wouldn't want clearer and more radiant skin? By making kimchi a regular part of your diet, your skin will receive a huge boost of nutrients to help it detoxify wastes, retain moisture and maintain an even skin tone. As discussed above, kimchi kicks inflammation to the curb like yesterday's trash. And inflammation is your skin's worst enemy, so anything that cools and soothes your skin from the inside out is worth its weight in gold!

High kimchi consumption (eaten at most meals) has been linked to lower incidence of eczema.

High kimchi consumption (eaten at most meals) has been linked to lower incidence of eczema (atopic dermatitis), while high consumption of processed foods and meat has been linked to a higher incidence of eczema, a skin disorder that's always puzzled the medical community as to its cause and how to heal it.[60] In animal studies, kimchi was shown to directly help promote healthy skin conditions.[61] In particular, one study found that 3-5 oz. (2-4 servings) of kimchi per day significantly reduced the incidence of atopic dermatitis in adults.[62] Kimchi does this by significantly altering our gut bacteria,[63] and using lactic acid bacteria topically can also improve this skin condition.[64] Finally, since acne is all about inflammation, we want to do everything we can to lower it by addressing the gut. Between the diet program I recommend in the next chapter and an increase in probiotics, kimchi works to heal dysbiosis and the intestinal issues that cause inflammation. Plus, with its anti-inflammatory ingredients like ginger and garlic, you'll be set for beautiful, radiant skin!

Kimchi works to heal dysbiosis and the intestinal issues that cause inflammation.

Acne or Mites?

Britney was a lovely 15-year-old teenager and had been battling cystic acne since she was twelve. The acne covered her forehead, cheeks and chest. Her mother Daphne had already taken her to five different dermatologists before coming to my office. Britney had tried their topical medications and skin care products, only to find that some worked for a little while and some made things worse. The doctors all told her mother that Britney needed to be on oral antibiotics, but she was reluctant to put her daughter on them because Britney had an allergic reaction to penicillin as a child. They came to see me because Britney was desperate to have clear skin.

When I looked closer with a high-powered magnification loupes (surgical glasses), I noticed that some areas on her face looked like true acne, but other areas did not. Many areas were red and inflamed but without pustules. I suspected she actually had demodex mites in her skin, and this didn't sit well with Britney or her mother. I wanted her to get it checked out under a microscope with her dermatologist, but they declined.

I mentioned that Britney's skin microbiome was completely out of balance. The pH of her skin was too acidic, causing acne breakouts. There was also the secondary issue of microscopic demodex mites living in her follicle and oil glands, causing more inflammation and irritation. We had to change her skin microbiome quickly, and to do that, I recommended we heal her gut first with The Kimchi Diet™. Skin problems often stem from an unhealthy gut.

When I mentioned to Britney that she'd have to start on The Kimchi Diet™, she was actually very happy with the treatment protocol. Her best friend Sunny was Korean and Britney loved going over for home-cooked meals and kimchi. My goal was to shift her internal and external skin microbiome, so that her immunity would be stronger and healthier from the inside out. I also changed her daily skin care routine and recommended that she needed to sweat more to open up her pores through exercise and steam facials.

Within two weeks on The Kimchi Diet™ and the all natural Purigenex® skin care regimen, Britney came back into the office with a huge smile on her face and gave me the biggest hug! The large cystic acne spots were healing and the discolorations and irritations were returning back to healthier-looking skin. There weren't any new acne spots either. Emotionally, she was feeling better about herself. Acne flare-ups triggered by her hormonal fluctuations (especially around her menstrual cycle) still affected her, so it took a total of three months to completely clear up.

Britney still eats kimchi daily and her acne scars are long gone, replaced by the beautiful vibrant skin she always dreamed of.

Cancer Prevention and Treatment

While preventing cancer necessitates a whole lifestyle of minimizing exposure to carcinogens, there are functional foods we can eat in order to help our body avoid its development. It's important not to smoke or drink and to avoid contact with toxic chemicals and pesticides in order to prevent cancer. But kimchi can also play a role in a healthy lifestyle change for cancer prevention. Park and Ju (2018) have shown how the "administration of kimchi may be helpful for lowering fecal pH and deactivation of hazardous enteric enzymes, which may result in maintaining good colon health and suppressing the formation of carcinogens, and eventually promote colon health and colorectal cancer prevention" and how even dead lactic acid bacteria from kimchi "prevented colitis and colon cancer in animal studies" (pg. 57).[65] This effect was increased with the use of Chinese pepper and organic cabbage. Their research also shows how kimchi prevents cancerous cell growth, but does not affect normal cells adversely. In other studies, kimchi has shown anti-cancer effects on both pancreatic and liver

Kimchi is a wonder food that should be part of a global revolution in healthful eating.

cancer cells, with a more pronounced effect on pancreatic cancer, which has historically been one of the more difficult to treat forms of cancer.[66] But kimchi's benefits don't stop there. Other researchers have seen it as not only having a role in cancer prevention, but also in treatment.[67] Kimchi is a wonder food that should be part of a global revolution in healthful eating.

Healthy Blood Pressure

You might think that with all the salt, kimchi might be bad for your blood pressure. Well, you're not alone. Recently, many Koreans have started to cut back on their kimchi consumption due to concerns with studies linking high kimchi consumption to hypertension. However, a recent study has shown this concern to be unwarranted as it was unable to find any definitive link between kimchi consumption and hypertension.[68] The scientists who did the study actually believe that the high level of potassium in kimchi is what helps to balance out the sodium, so there's no negative effect on blood pressure. So please feel free to enjoy your kimchi every day without concern about your blood pressure, but just to be sure, ask your doctor first!

In fact, the many vitamins, minerals, enzymes and phytochemicals that are found in kimchi will help you to achieve and maintain healthy blood pressure.

Now that we've learned all about kimchi history and its almost endless health benefits, the only thing left to do is start making and eating kimchi every day. It couldn't be a more simple lifestyle change to make, but it's one that can truly bring about life-changing results for you and your family.

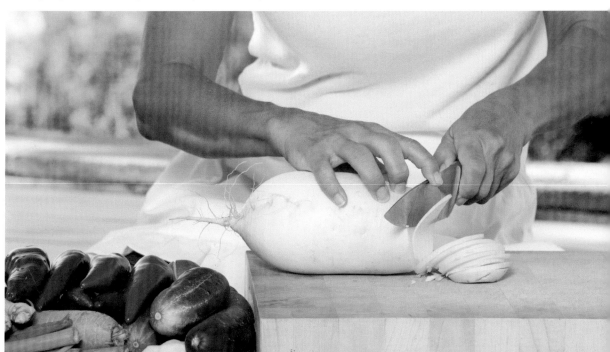

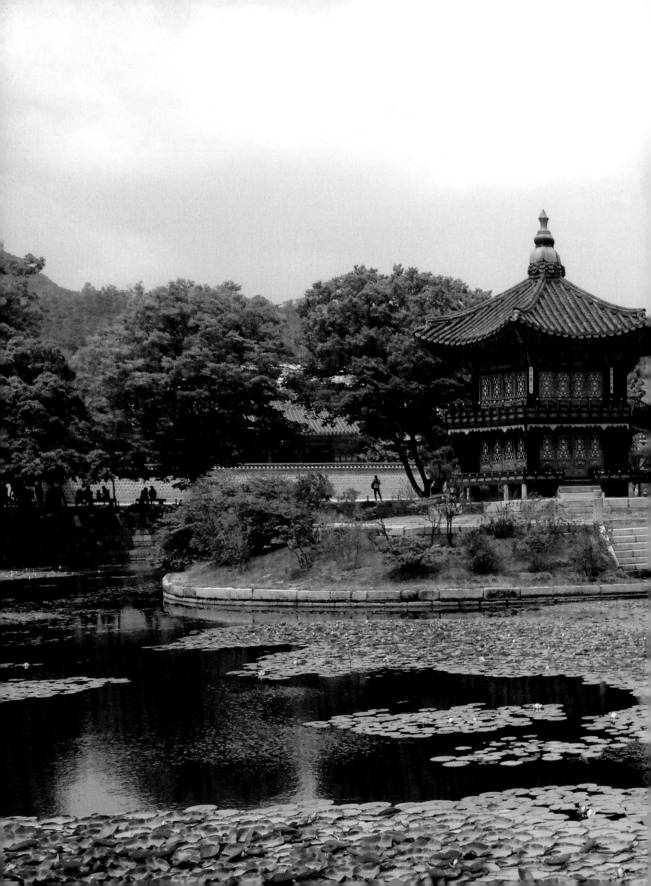

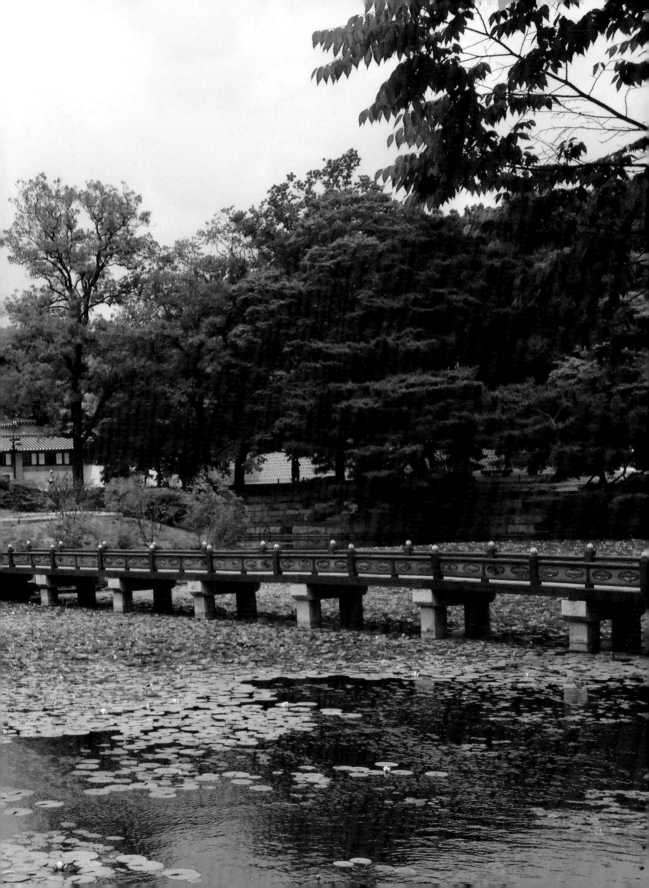

Chapter 3

The Kimchi Diet™

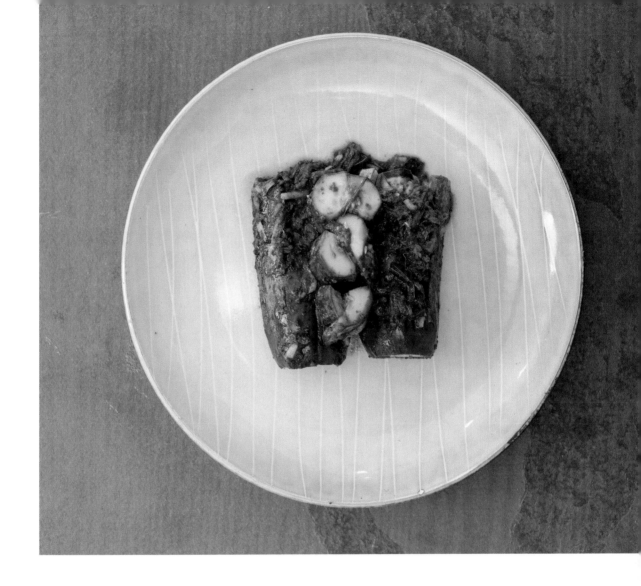

Alright, it's almost time to start making, storing and most importantly: eating kimchi! In this chapter, I detail an 8-week plan with specific recommendations for which types of kimchi to start with, when to make each batch, and when to eat them for optimal taste and a good dose of beneficial probiotics.

After many years of introducing kimchi into my patients' diets, I discovered that there are specific recipes that work better than others at each step of the process. It's why I've set up my Kimchi Diet™ the way I have—to give the best results. The truth is, more often than not, newbie kimchi enthusiasts immediately start eating napa cabbage kimchi, since that's what is most available commercially. Doing so, they often end up disappointed, with a strong case of gas and bloating! It's why I start with "simpler" types of kimchi and have you work up to napa kimchi.

For that reason, it's important to remember that eating kimchi will increase the lactic acid bacteria in your gut, and in the beginning it may feel a bit like a war zone—with good bacteria fighting the bad. Be patient. The purpose of The Kimchi Diet™ is to be consistent and feed your gut with the good lactic acid bacteria, so ultimately they outshine the rest. Following the plan in this chapter allows you to have a steady supply of kimchi for eight weeks—each one timed for maximum benefit and deliciousness!

Remember, The Kimchi Diet™ is not about counting calories, starvation, or crash dieting. It's about adding fermented kimchi into your life daily.

Remember, The Kimchi Diet™ is not about counting calories, starvation, or crash dieting. It's about adding fermented kimchi into your life daily. And you can add it to pretty much any diet—vegan, Mediterranean, paleo, keto, macrobiotic and so forth. With that being said, we can't ignore the scientific fact that if you start with a healthful plan of eating together with The Kimchi Diet™, it'll make a much bigger difference in relieving your symptoms. That's why I'm including my guide to healthful eating, so you have the best chance of truly thriving on The Kimchi Diet™.

Preparation Phase: A Commitment to Healthful Eating

As you begin The Kimchi Diet™, it's important to eat as healthily as possible. Just think about it: kimchi may be a very powerful superfood, but no superfood alone can possibly have its full effects if your body is having to spend its energy processing bad food. Unfortunately, the standard American diet is chock-full of foods that are difficult for the body to deal with. From processed foods to refined sugars to deep fried foods, sometimes it seems our whole diet is meant to put a stress on the system. These foods may not produce a noticeable effect if you only eat them once a year. But if you eat them every week, they can produce inflammatory responses—as if your body thinks it's sick! Even though you may not have a full-blown anaphylactic or IgE reaction, the body slowly becomes inflamed and spends its valuable resources trying to "fight" these food stressors, instead of spending all its vital energy on mental function, hormone regulation, pumping blood, and so forth.

In the course of thirty years, working with patients suffering from allergies, irritable bowel syndrome, chronic fatigue and more, I've developed an Anti-Inflammatory Nutrition Plan (check the Resource section on page 153 to get the full list of foods to eat and ones to avoid) that's meant to help reduce inflammation quickly and make the body feel vibrant, so it can run at its optimal capacity. It's the one I detail in *The 7-Day Allergy Makeover*, the one that helped my son, Cody to overcome his life-threatening allergies, and the same one (with some key additions) that I used to help my recovery from brain injury, as I talk about in *The Mighty Mito*. This is not a crash diet, cleanse, detox or quick fix. It's a nutrition plan to follow for the *rest of your life*, because it embodies the best of healthy eating from my clinical experience and research over the years. So even if you haven't read those books, I want to give you the condensed version of my Anti-Inflammatory Nutrition Plan here.

The Anti-Inflammatory Nutrition Plan

To begin with, the simple rule to follow is this: **eat whole, natural, unprocessed and organic foods**. Vegetables, fruits, free-range meat, nuts, seeds and ancient grains like quinoa and amaranth are all great options. In general, try to fill half your plate with veggies (this is where the kimchi comes in!), a quarter of it with protein (beans, meat) and a quarter of it with healthful grains. Top it off with good fats like olive oil or avocado. Just following this one simple rule can change so much for so many Americans!

Beyond that, there are four food groups that I recommend eliminating completely from your diet: *gluten products, dairy, sugars* (including alcohol) and *artificial, highly processed ingredients*. In my clinical practice and medical research, I've found that many people are extremely sensitive to these foods, often without knowing it. These foods often cause hidden inflammatory reactions in the gut—leading to inflammation and increased permeability in the gut lining, known as "leaky gut syndrome." Furthermore, everything from brain fog, energy crashes and rashes all the way up to acid reflux, bloating, diarrhea and vomiting have been traced back to the consumption of certain foods in this group among some of my patients. Let me briefly detail what to cut out and most importantly, why.

Gluten Products

Gluten is what makes bread and wheat "chewy" and is especially difficult for our digestive system to process, due to the high levels of *fructans*—long chains of fructose molecules. Not to mention that most commercially produced wheat is sprayed with an herbicide made of glyphosate, possibly the worst herbicide out there. Therefore, please eliminate:

- Wheat (whole and white)
- Oats (unless specified as gluten-free)
- Barley
- Rye
- Spelt
- Kamut

- Bread and bagels
- Donuts
- Pasta

Nowadays, you can find many gluten-free foods, from pizza crusts to pasta to bread. Make sure that these are made of quinoa, brown rice, wild rice, corn or amaranth. Still it's best to limit your consumption of these foods, as they can also lead to inflammation. You might try replacing them with a vegetable like cauliflower, which can often work well with recipes that call for grains.

Dairy Products

Along with the gluten-free revolution, the dairy-free revolution has hit the United States hard in the last decade. The majority of the population after the age of five is lactose intolerant due to the lack of lactase enzyme production by the brush borders of the small intestine. Without the ability to digest lactose, people's bodies are irritated by the undigested sugar in milk. It can cause an overgrowth of bacteria and yeast, triggering irritable bowel symptoms such as gas, bloating, cramping and diarrhea. As mentioned above, leaky gut syndrome is caused by the inflammatory response of too much sugar. Dairy can contribute to this syndrome as well.

Traditional Korean cuisine is both gluten-free and dairy-free.

Traditional Korean cuisine is both gluten-free *and* dairy-free. If you go to a Korean restaurant, you will see some foods made with wheat or milk, but these are due to the more recent history of Westernization. 99% of Korean food is still based on gluten-free and dairy-free recipes.

Eliminating dairy products means cutting out anything made with cow's, sheep's or goat's milk.

- Milk
- Cheese
- Ice Cream
- Yogurt
- Sour Cream
- Cream Cheese
- Dairy Salad Dressings or Sauces

Instead, try the many unsweetened alternatives made from rice, almond, walnut (my favorite), hazelnut, coconut or hemp. Some people are reactive to soy products, so I can't recommend soy milk for everyone. Many people mistake eggs for a dairy product, but they should not be put in this category. Eggs are a great source of protein—although once again—many of my patients have been sensitive to them. If you're not, I certainly encourage you to eat eggs from pasture-raised organic chickens.

Sugars

With all the problems that we face from diabetes and Alzheimer's, it's no wonder that sugar is at the top of many doctors' "Do Not Eat" list. But as the market gets flooded with supposedly more healthful alternatives, many people are confused about what's okay and what's not okay to consume.

Here's my simple formula: do your best to not eat any sweetener, even if it's all natural, like honey or agave. Sugar and refined carbs (like white rice) spike the blood sugar and lead to energy crashes and brain fog, or if consumed in high enough quantities, insulin resistance. That's right, foods like white pasta or white bread are almost entirely simple sugars at the end of the day, so I recommend eliminating them. Cutting out sugar is one of the single best things you can do for your health.

Now, with that said, you'll notice that sugar can be one of the ingredients in kimchi recipes. So why is that? The sugar is something added—usually one teaspoon—for the lactic acid bacteria to feed on. Once they feed on it, however, you are not actually ingesting the sugar, but rather the byproducts of the fermentation process itself. The point of this sugar is not to increase calories, but simply to allow the lactic acid bacteria to grow, and it does provide a slightly sweeter taste. Once again, the sugar in kimchi is completely optional. With that said, you'll want to avoid:

- Sugar (White, Brown, Raw, Turbinado)
- Honey
- Molasses
- Evaporated Cane Juice
- Agave Nectar
- Coconut Sugar
- Date Sugar
- Maple Syrup

- White rice
- White bread and pasta (Contains Gluten)
- Alcohol

Some monk fruit and erythritol sweeteners are good options. Stevia is ok too. Just make sure they have *nothing* else added. Some even have lactose—which is a dairy product, so beware!

Food Additives and Highly Processed Ingredients

Finally, we get to food additives, which really aren't foods at all. These are chemicals used to make food look better, stay preserved longer, or supposedly taste better. Some, like high fructose corn syrup, come from natural sources but have no nutritional value. There's no reason to eat these, and considering what a toxic burden they add to the body, there's almost nothing you can do to improve your health more than refrain from eating the following:

- Aspartame (Nutrasweet®, blue packet)
- Sucralose (Splenda®, yellow packet)
- Saccharin (Sweet 'N Low®, pink packet)
- High Fructose Corn Syrup
- MSG (monosodium glutamate)
- Food Coloring (red, blue, yellow dyes)
- Nitrites (sausage, deli meats)
- Sulfites (wine, beer, deli food)
- BHA (pork sausages, chips, instant tea, packaged food)
- Butylates or BHT (butter, vegetable oils, margarine)
- Benzoates (fruit juices, ketchup, tea, coffee)
- Hydrogenated Oils (margarine, vegetable shortening, packaged snacks)

In addition to these foods, I recommend that people who are especially prone to allergies or have digestive issues consider cutting out eggs, peanuts, mushrooms and soy products. You can then try reintroducing them one by one to see if you have any reactions. If not, feel free to enjoy them in your daily life. For more information on the Anti-Inflammatory Nutrition Plan, check out *The 7-Day Allergy Makeover* or the Resource section.

For Those with Irritable Bowel Syndrome or Gut Issues

If you've been diagnosed with irritable bowel syndrome or often experience bloating, gas, poor digestion or constipation, you should modify the above diet to help your gut bacteria "reset." Often, these symptoms are the result of an overload of what are known as fermentable carbohydrates—namely, foods that bacteria in the gut help our body to process. In addition, when you eat too many fermentable carbohydrates or don't have enough helpful gut bacteria, this process can become less efficient, resulting in an overload of gas—which is a byproduct of bacterial fermentation. So what's the way out of this conundrum?

I recommend the Anti-Inflammatory Nutrition Plan described above, but with a twist. You also want to reduce your intake of fermentable carbohydrates, often known as FODMAP foods. This acronym stands for Fermentable Oligosaccharides, Disaccharides,

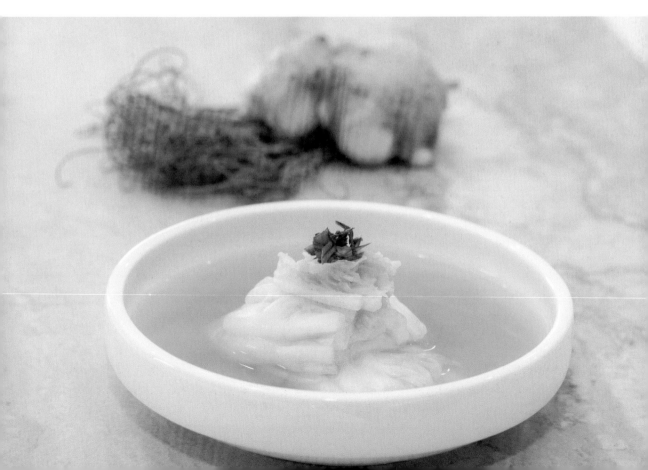

Monosaccharides and Polyols, which basically means the types of carbohydrates that our body processes through fermentation. These sugars need to be processed through fermentation in the gut, since the human body does not produce the enzymes to break them down. If too many FODMAP foods are eaten, especially when there is an overgrowth of bad bacteria or fungi, then irritable bowel symptoms may appear. Reducing the intake of fermentable carbohydrates in the beginning of The Kimchi Diet™ will calm your gut down, improve your energy and minimize other symptoms.

While the lists below are not exhaustive, they give you an idea of which foods to avoid. For a more complete list of foods to eat and foods to avoid, I've combined the Anti-Inflammatory Nutrition Plan and FODMAP-Free Diet to make *The Ultimate Wellness for Life Food List*, which is available in the Resource section on page 153.

The FODMAP Foods

The following are FODMAP foods, and ones that I have all my patients eliminate as part of the standard Anti-Inflammatory Nutrition Plan:

- Sugars
- Alcohol
- Gluten Grains
- Dairy Products

Additionally, there are many healthful foods that are high in fermentable carbohydrates which you'll need to eliminate temporarily from your diet if you experience IBS symptoms:

- Beans
- Soy Products
- Cabbage
- Cruciferous Vegetables (Broccoli, Cauliflower)
- Artichokes
- Asparagus
- Apples

- Cherries
- Pears
- Watermelon
- Apricots
- Prunes

These are all normally great foods to eat (with the possible exception of soy for some people) and very healthy. However, if you have a bacterial overgrowth, the excess bacteria will feed on these foods and produce gas and bloating, since the body lacks the enzymes needed to break them down.

Cut them out of your diet for four to six weeks to reduce the bacterial overgrowth, depending on when you start feeling better. Then *slowly* introduce them back in to your diet one at a time. Remember that fermentable carbohydrates are *not* to be eliminated forever. You just want to limit them for a short time if you have a bacterial overgrowth and irritable bowel symptoms. Consider this part of your gut healing program.

I've intentionally designed The Kimchi Diet™ to start with lower-FODMAP foods (like cucumbers) and end up with higher-FODMAP foods like cabbage, to help accommodate everyone. Sometimes even a person with a healthy gut can be a bit overwhelmed if they start eating cabbage every single day! The good news is that there's almost nothing better you can do to help your irritable bowel symptoms than eat kimchi, as its helpful probiotics will work to digest FODMAP foods.

There's almost nothing better you can do to help your irritable bowel symptoms than eat kimchi, as its helpful probiotics will work to digest FODMAP foods.

Although I'm asking you to take inflammatory foods out of your diet for faster results, I'd like to emphasis again that The Kimchi Diet™ is about *adding kimchi* to whatever diet you're on, whether it's meat and potatoes or a vegan diet.

This is not about deprivation, but rather health by addition.

If it's too difficult for you or your family to eliminate all of these inflammatory foods, then take just one of the following groups out of your diet completely: gluten grains, sugars or dairy foods. After you start seeing positive changes, it may be easier to get rid of the next food offender and feel more motivated to make true lifelong changes. While the ideal nutrition program might be sugar-free, gluten-free, dairy-free, organic and free of food additives, it may take your family a while to get there—and that's okay. True health is a long-term process!

The 8-Week Kimchi Diet™

Here begins our 8-week journey into the magical world of kimchi. What I suggest below is the plan I've developed over the years for introducing my patients to this wonder food in order to minimize stomach distress and to ensure a steady stream of new kimchi tastes and flavors. It's helped to reduce allergies, clear up acne, produce weight loss, reduce pain and inflammation and increase energy and brain clarity.

In addition, the magic of The Kimchi Diet™ is in the optimal levels of lactic acid bacteria you'll be ingesting daily. You can always modify it, try new vegetables or add new varieties of kimchi to your meals. But by starting on this 8-week plan, you'll have a great head start when it comes to transforming your gut biome and your health with the power of kimchi.

Although I'm providing you with a timeline schedule for The Kimchi Diet™ 8-week plan, don't feel that you have to follow it exactly as it's laid out. Some of my patients need more time to revive their gut and may take sixteen weeks instead of eight—and if that's the case for you, no problem! Move at your own pace, as you know best how fast you can move from one phase to the next. Actually, your gut will tell you!

To maximize kimchi health benefits, the most important schedule you want to follow is eating the right type of kimchi from the start.

To maximize kimchi health benefits, the most important schedule you want to follow is eating the right type of kimchi from the start, and in a sequential manner from Phase 1 to Phase 4. The amount of time between each phase is not as important as eating kimchi daily is for gut healing success!

As I describe each phase of The Kimchi Diet™ below, I recommend that you also flip to The Kimchi Diet™ Recipe chapter starting on page 127 to familiarize yourself with each type of kimchi, plus there are a lot of instructional images that will be super helpful. Visuals make it so much easier to process!

Here's a quick overview of the entire plan.

Quick Summary of The Kimchi Diet™ Timeline

Phase 1: Days 1–14

Day 1: Make Cucumber Kimchi.

Day 3–4: Start eating 2 to 3 pieces from one cucumber kimchi floret daily.

Day 7–8: Work up to eating an entire cucumber kimchi floret daily.

Day 8: Make baby bok choy, mustard greens, radish tops or beet tops kimchi.

Day 8–14: Continue to eat 1 cucumber kimchi floret daily.

Phase 2: Days 14–28

Day 14–21: Finish off the cucumber kimchi and start eating 1 tablespoon of the Phase 2 kimchi of your choice (baby bok choy, mustard greens, radish tops or beet tops), working up to two tablespoons per day.

Day 21: Make root vegetable kimchi (radish, daikon, turnip or rutabaga kimchi).

Day 21–28: Continue eating Phase 2 kimchi.

Phase 3: Days 28–42

Day 28: Continue to finish off the Phase 2 kimchi, and start eating one to two tablespoons of the root vegetable kimchi (radish, daikon, turnip or rutabaga kimchi).

Day 28: Make the napa cabbage kimchi.

Day 28–42: Continue to eat 2–3 tablespoons of both Phase 2 and Phase 3 kimchi daily.

Phase 4: Days 42–56 and Beyond

Day 42: Eat one to two tablespoons of napa cabbage kimchi and watch out for symptoms.

Day 42–56: Continue eating the Phase 2 & Phase 3 kimchi, (whatever is left) and continue incorporating napa cabbage kimchi into your diet. Work up to eating 4 tablespoons of kimchi per day.

Four tablespoons is about a quarter cup of kimchi, which means you'll be ingesting over 60 billion CFUs of lactic acid bacteria per day!

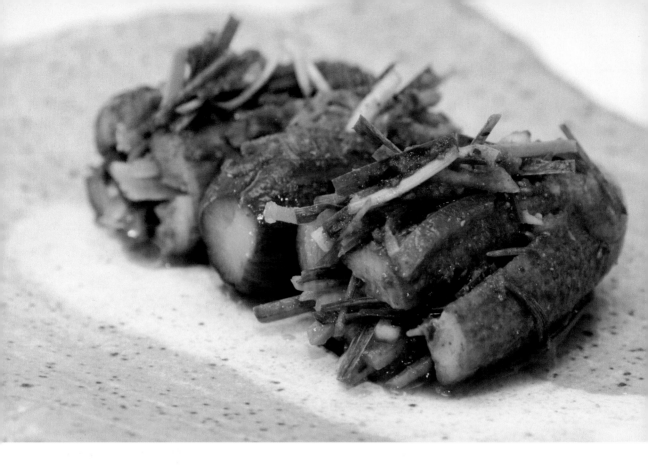

On **Day 1** (or before), be sure you have all the appropriate Kimchi Tools:

- Sharp Knife
- Cutting Board
- Large Mixing Bowl
- Colander
- Fruit Grater
- Gloves and Apron (for handling the red pepper powder and kimchi paste)
- Glass Jars (Mason jars or airtight containers)
- Earthenware Containers (optional, if you prefer to glass)

You'll then need to go to the store and get the core ingredients for kimchi: solar sea salt, garlic, ginger, coarse red pepper powder, Asian pears (Bosc pears are fine), Fuji apples and spring onions. This week you'll be making Cucumber Kimchi (see page 128), a very easy, light kimchi that you can start eating *within days*. So buy some cucumbers as well. You can make it as mild or spicy as you prefer, but do remember that many of the beneficial bacteria and health benefits of kimchi come from the red pepper powder, so if possible, try to add it. I find spicy kimchi absolutely irresistible!

Although Cucumber Kimchi can be eaten as soon as it's made, as many Koreans do, to maximize on the health benefits of the LAB and phytonutrients, allow the magic of fermentation to take place first!

Beginning on **Day 3** or **4**, take one floret out from the bottom of the jar to ensure you're getting the good bacteria in the juices.

Peel each cucumber leaf away from the stalk and cut it up into small bite size pieces. Eat only three to four pieces once a day, as a side dish or salad with your lunch or dinner.

At this stage, a low level of lactic acid bacteria has been established, and adding Cucumber Kimchi into your diet will be easy.

Top your roasted chicken with a piece of cucumber kimchi, add it to veggies to improve the flavor, or you can serve it over quinoa or inside a taco. It even goes well with scrambled eggs!

What you'll notice during the first few days of fermentation is that the kimchi will still taste a bit like seasoned raw cucumbers, but within a week as it deepens the fermentation process, you will be delighted with a tangy, slightly sweet, robust, pungent flavor! That's the bacteria doing its job.

Enjoy the progression of tastes, as it goes from mild to fully ripe and you will refine your kimchi taste buds in no time!

Starting on **Day 8**, make either Bok Choy (most available in stores), Beet Tops, Mustard Green Tops or Radish Tops Kimchi (page 134). Again, mild or spicy is okay. You will not eat this kimchi right away, but instead let it ferment for a week before digging in. Then on day fourteen you can start enjoying them, right as the Cucumber Kimchi comes to an end.

As the Cucumber Kimchi ferments gradually in the refrigerator for the next two weeks, the LAB will continuously grow in number, ultimately to a level of up to 1 billion CFU's per gram of kimchi.

Work your way up to eating one whole cucumber floret twice a day by the end of Day **10 to 14**.

It's best to eat Cucumber Kimchi within three weeks of making it, because it loses its crunchy texture and can become super sour after that. It will not "go bad" even if it's a month old, but just know that the texture will become soft and mushy. Cucumber kimchi juice is still good for consumption—it's amazingly delicious and full of probiotics.

One tablespoon of kimchi a day will keep the doctor away!

By the way, if you can't eat spicy foods, no worries! Kimchi can be made without the red pepper. In fact, for the first 1700 years kimchi was made without red pepper. At the end of each recipe in Chapter 5, I've added special notes on how to make the recipe without the red pepper powder. Without the red pepper, the fermentation process will be quicker and you may need to pop it into the refrigerator sooner, maybe 6 to 8 hours after the initial room temperature fermentation. You'll also need to eat the non-spicy kimchi you make faster than the spicy ones.

During Phase 1, don't be alarmed if you start to feel that something is definitely stirring up in your intestines. You'll be happy to know that there's a "bug war" going on in your gut for the first few weeks, but in your favor. The LAB found in the kimchi naturally helps to eliminate unhealthy bacteria in your digestive tract, and there will be a short phase of struggle for microbial hierarchy. But the good guys will be the king of the hill at the end. However, if you experience excess bloating, gas, burping, abdominal cramping or diarrhea after incorporating cucumber kimchi into your diet, I recommend you stop for a few days or when the symptoms have calmed down and then reintroduce it back into your diet, but only eat half of the amount daily, or eat it every other day.

KIMCHI TIP: How to Get Rid of Kimchi Breath?

Some people notice a slightly garlicky odor to their breath after eating kimchi. Well, I've got that one solved as well. My secret is *ginger*!

I discovered this kimchi breath cure many years ago while I was doing research for one of my Purigenex™ skin care products, Age Reverse Serum. One key

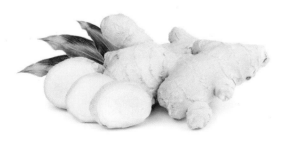

ingredient I wanted to add to the formula was liposomal glutathione, a super antioxidant and anti-aging cosmeceutical, but it had a very heavy sulfur note.

I must have tested over fifty different natural fragrances to neutralize the sulfur smell and finally found the note that masked it—ginger.

Ever since, I began to drink ginger tea right after eating kimchi, which means pretty much after every meal. I even carry a small bottle of organic ginger powder in my purse just in case we go to the local Korean restaurant. Not only will it freshen your breath, you'll also get some of the amazing health benefits of ginger, as it's an antioxidant, anti-inflammatory, a sugar balancer and more!

Kimchi Breath Cure

Add 1/4 teaspoon of ginger in 10 oz. of hot or cold water, dissolve and drink after eating any type of kimchi. This ginger drink will help with garlic and onion breath too!

Phase 2: Days 14–28

By **Day 14**, you may have eaten most of the Cucumber Kimchi, and if it's overly ripe—that is—if it tastes sour and has lost its crunchiness, you can compost or discard it. If it still tastes great, continue eating small amounts of it and begin to add the Mustard Greens or Radish Tops Kimchi into your diet.

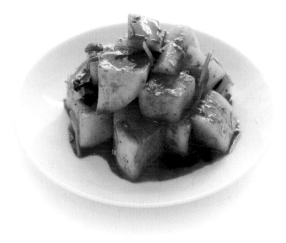

Your second batch of kimchi should be ripe enough to be consumed on **Day 14**, after just one week of fermentation. Begin with one tablespoon per day, with lunch or dinner. As the days go by, if you feel good and your body and intestinal tract allow it (no allergic reactions, bloating, gas or indigestion), then have a tablespoon of the kimchi twice per day—one with lunch and one with dinner.

For the next two weeks (**Days 14–28**), continue to ingest up to two tablespoons of the Mustard Greens or Radish Tops Kimchi. The kimchi will be fully ripe and the level of kimchi microbiome will be optimal. Sourness should be minimal at this point.

Starting on **Day 21**, make a root vegetable kimchi: Daikon, Turnip, Radish or Rutabaga Kimchi that's to be eaten a week later: **Day 28** or so (138). My favorite is Korean Radish and my second favorite is Daikon (more narrow)—but be sure to experiment and find your own! Most kimchi can take about a week or two to be ready, with cucumber and some lighter vegetables being the exception.

As mentioned, continue eating two tablespoons of Mustard Greens, Beet Tops, Bok Choy or Radish Tops Kimchi per day and if you feel your gut is ready to be introduced to another type of kimchi, then add one tablespoon of the Root Vegetable Kimchi per day around **Day 28**. If you experience discomfort in any way, you can always go back to two tablespoons of Phase 1 or Phase 2 kimchi per day. The Kimchi Diet™ is a personalized plan that's to be implemented at your own pace for your own health needs.

Phase 3: Days 28–42

The Radish Kimchi or other hard root vegetable will last you for the next two week to four weeks. Continue eating two tablespoons a day from **Day 28–42** with your lunch and dinner. These root vegetables can actually last for four to six weeks or even longer, depending on how much you make and consume. Radish Kimchi juice is considered medicinal as a diarrhea or constipation remedy. I have two or three bottles of the leftover juice in my fridge and periodically I take a tablespoon here and there because of the refreshing taste and the lactic acid bacteria.

By now you've been inoculating your digestive tract with billions of lactic bacteria daily. Remember, one gram of kimchi has about one billion CFUs (colony forming units) of helpful bacteria, so you're on quite a roll. Many people begin to notice changes in their bodies around this time. You may feel different in your gut, a bit lighter, less bloated, less anxious or like you have more energy. Don't worry if not. It can take some time to gauge a difference, especially if you have a depleted gut microbiome. Starting on **Day 28**, you'll want to make Napa Cabbage Kimchi (page 141) to be eaten on the sixth week of The Kimchi Diet™. This is the kimchi that most people think of when they visualize kimchi and it's my personal favorite. There's something about the crunchy cabbage, the spice, and the garlic and ginger that wins me over every time. This one needs a little more time than the other kimchis, not because it takes more time to ferment, but because the extra time allows the LAB to predigest the napa cabbage longer, reducing the fermentable carbohydrate levels. This will minimize symptoms of gas and bloating.

Phase 4: Days 42–56 and Beyond

Napa Kimchi is the litmus test to see if your gut microbiome is optimal. Start eating it on **Day 42**, just one tablespoon at a time. If your microbiome is still imbalanced, you'll have a lot of gas, bloating, and many bouts of bowel movements and even loose stool. If so, back off on the Napa Cabbage Kimchi and continue with the other kimchi. Just remake the Cucumber Kimchi for a fast treat or go back to Mustard Greens or Radishes—your choice.

However, if all goes well, you should keep eating the Napa Kimchi—it's perhaps the most potent variety for helping to restore the gut microbiome. Eat one to two tablespoons for at least the next two weeks, until **Day 56**. By that time, check in with yourself. How do you feel now compared to when you started? Do you feel more energetic, alert and in a better mood? Have you lost weight or do you feel more comfortable in your body? These are all signs to recognize that The Kimchi Diet™ is working!

If you feel really good, try to slowly build up to four tablespoons of kimchi per day, splitting it up between two meals. Four tablespoons is about a quarter cup of kimchi, so you would be ingesting over 60 billion CFUs of diverse lactic acid bacteria per day.

But The Kimchi Diet™ doesn't end after eight weeks! Incorporating kimchi into your meals every day is simply one of the best things you can do for your family. I encourage you to have some Napa Cabbage or Radish Kimchi on hand at all times. Plus, if you're out of fresh vegetables for your next meal, there's always kimchi available to help you reach your veggie quota for the day!

I usually make a new batch of kimchi every two weeks and have many different bottles of kimchi at various stages of fermentation in my kimchi refrigerator, and some bottles that are three months old, yum!

That's part of the joy of kimchi—you can make it with veggies you like and have it ready to go in just a week or two with no cooking and almost no hassle.

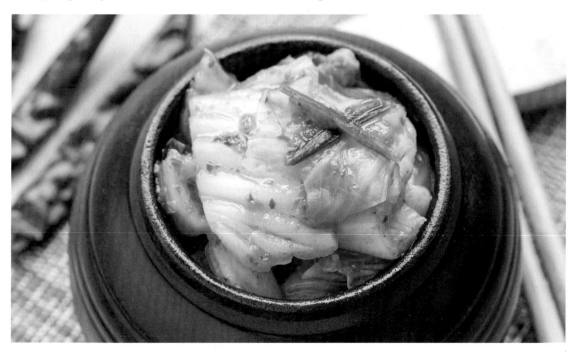

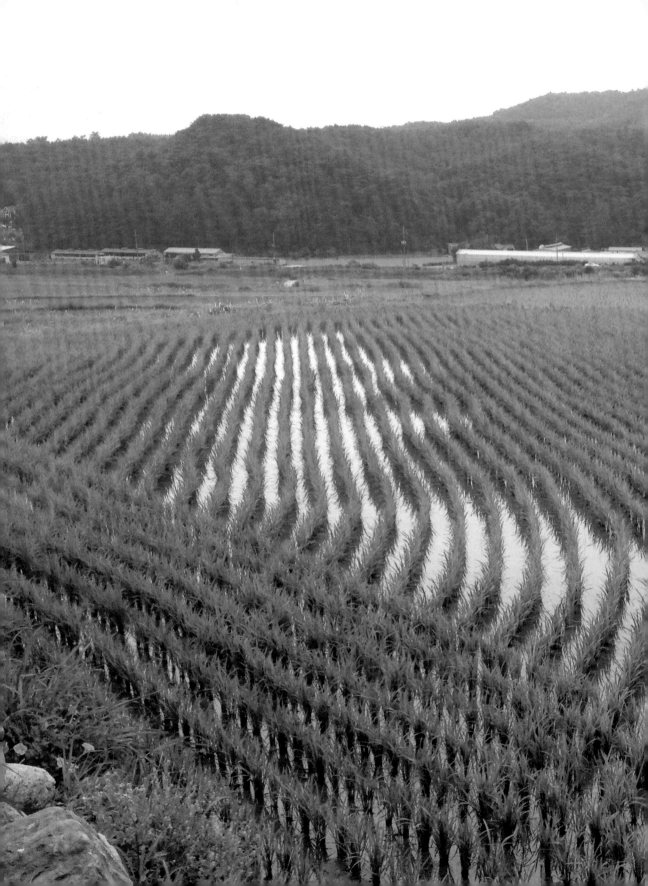

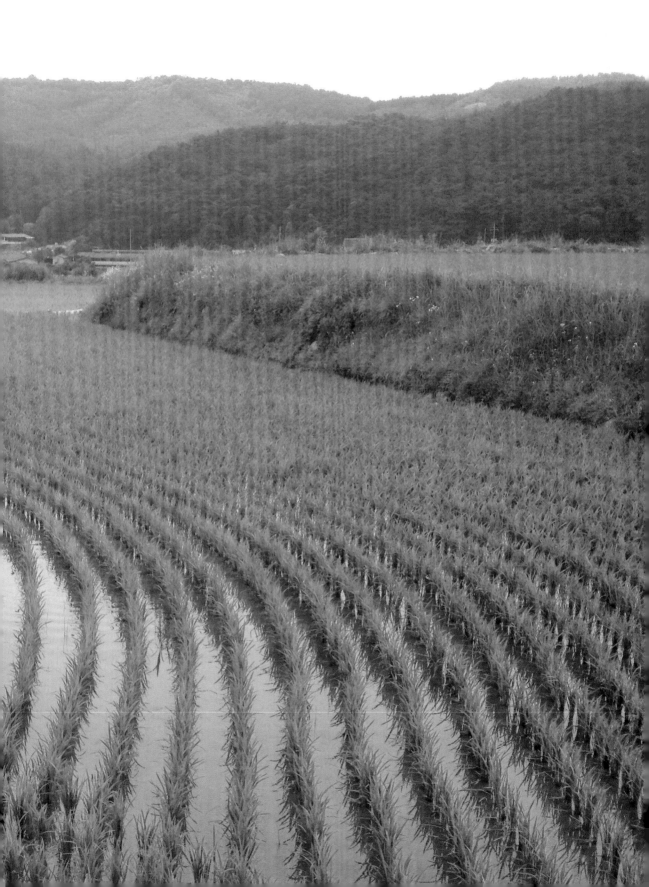

Chapter 4

How to Make Kimchi
An Overview

Now that we have The Kimchi Diet™ plan all laid out, it's time for an overview on how to make kimchi. This chapter offers some general steps and tips for kimchi preparation, although you'll find the details on how to make specific types of kimchi in the recipe section of the book, Chapter 5.

If you've ever had a bite of kimchi, and I mean real, *It's truly a full-body,* authentic, traditional kimchi made by a Korean family (not the *sensorial experience.* American versions that are now available in the health food stores and farmers' markets), you'll know that it's truly a full-body, sensorial experience. To this day, whenever I even think of kimchi my mouth immediately salivates—truly a classic case of a Pavlovian response!

All my senses get fully activated as if I'm eating a big bite of it: the bubbly sweet and sour taste, the pungent smell of fermented vegetables, the aroma of garlic, ginger and red pepper, the cool and crisp feel in the mouth, the crunchy sound of each bite, and the bright Technicolor of red, white and green of the vegetables, all so vividly clear.

It's this culture of kimchi, passed down from mother to daughter over dozens of generations that I hope to bring to you in the next two chapters, so that you'll not only

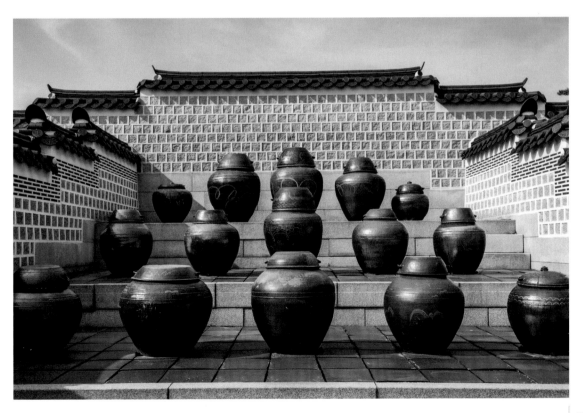

get the great health benefits of kimchi, but you'll enjoy it exactly as my mother and grandmother before her intended it to be eaten. I want you to experience that full-body sense of contentment that we Koreans call siwonhan-mat, an untranslatable term that means a "relief from pressure" or "physical calibration", specifically after eating a delicious meal. If you've ever gone to a Korean restaurant or to a Korean friend's house and had a meal, you'll know this feeling well. I hope that my grandmother's, mother's and my own kimchi recipes will give you all of this and more.

The Culture of Making Kimchi

There's an ancient Korean proverb that says something like this: "The best kimchi flavor depends on oemoni's sohn, or "mother's hand." And in our extended family, *halmeoni's*

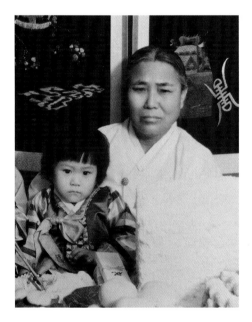

sohn (grandmother's hand) made the best kimchi. The honor was given to the elder, of course, as elders are treasured in all indigenous cultures as the wise and respected ones. My grandmother lived for 104 years on this planet, and I know kimchi had something to do with it. My mother is 87 and counting at the time of this publication and I'm doing everything I can to follow in these beautiful women's footsteps.

Speaking of elder generations, kimchi recipes were passed down the matriarchal lineage, and my mother was taught at a very early age how to make kimchi, not by any precise measurements, but by using her human senses: touch, sound, sight, taste and smell. I urge you not to think of your food, and kimchi in particular, as mere "fuel" for your body, but a complete sensory experience. Many Americans take very little time observing their food before chowing down—often at a very rapid speed—which can cause indigestion, bloating and cramping. I highly suggest you take the time to make eating kimchi a more mindful experience. Not only will you enjoy it more, but taking more time to eat your food also helps you to eat less overall and gives your body more time to digest it. Take the time to appreciate it aesthetically, all its flavors, smells, colors and textures, and you'll be rewarded.

Touch is used to check the freshness of the cabbage. As I washed the vegetables, my mother taught me to make sure the slippery film was washed off each napa leaf. My mother would say it had to "sound" clean: "*sak, sak.*" Fifty years ago, parasites were easily transmitted through food, so it was doubly important for them to be squeaky clean. My mother said the sound will tell you when it's clean. Washing the cabbage under water should be "sak sak" clean.

My halmeoni taught my mother that the sight of the beautiful vibrant colors of kimchi was important for our mind and appetite: the color combination of green, red, white and yellow in particular. There's the green onion or buchu namul, garlic shoots, and the bright red intensity of the red pepper flakes. White was the ideal color of cabbage and radish (my favorite) and yellow was for the fresh and aromatic couple, ginger and garlic. Ginger and garlic are key ingredients in making kimchi. Not only do they have ancient medicinal properties, but they also carry the natural microbes necessary to promote the fermentation process. My mantra is: "You can always make kimchi as long as you have ginger, garlic, sea salt and a vegetable." Everything else is an added plus and only contributes to the flavors and visual pleasure of the dish.

My mantra is: "You can always make kimchi as long as you have ginger, garlic, sea salt and a vegetable."

What You Need: The Basics

Before we start making kimchi, it's important to know everything you'll need and what the actual process of making kimchi consists of. Fortunately, it's very easy and not too time consuming, so the health benefits are really worth the effort you put in.

First, remember the basic kitchenware outlined in Chapter 3:

- Sharp Knife
- Cutting Board
- Large Mixing Bowl
- Colander
- Fruit Grater
- Gloves (for handling the red pepper powder)
- Glass Jars (Mason jars or airtight containers)
- Earthenware Containers (optional,

  if you prefer to glass)

You'll also need to check the recipe that you make each week before you do your grocery shopping. For instance, in week one of The Kimchi Diet™, you'll be making Cucumber Kimchi (see page 128), so you'll need to add cucumbers to the shopping list.

However, there are some ingredients that nearly every kimchi recipe requires and that you'll want to have on hand every week. They are:

- Vegetables
- Solar Sea Salt
- Garlic
- Ginger
- Green Onions
- Asian Pear or Fuji Apple
- Red Pepper Coarse Powder

    (optional but very healthful)

Superstar Ingredients

It's worth highlighting four ingredients in particular, because they're so important: solar sea salt, red pepper coarse powder, garlic and ginger. They're what I call the "superstar ingredients", because they make kimchi taste exceptional, and each one also has specific functional superpowers! So before moving on, let's go into a bit of detail on the benefits of these superstars.

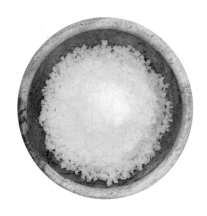

It's very important to get solar sea salt, not only for the growth of lactic acid bacteria in kimchi, but also for the quality and flavor.

Solar Sea Salt

Solar sea salt is produced naturally by solar evaporation in salt pans and has much higher concentrations of beneficial minerals such as magnesium, calcium and potassium than other types of salt. Please note that it's *very* important to get **solar sea salt**, not only for the growth of lactic acid bacteria in kimchi, but also for the quality and flavor. Sensory analysis indicates that the texture and crunchiness in kimchi will be not be as optimal if refined salt or table salt is used. In addition, some sea salts are naturally high in sodium chloride and low in other healthy minerals. I can't imagine making kimchi with table salt, which can be fortified with iodine. I don't consider kimchi made with it as worthy of eating. I may be biased, but I like Korean sea salt the best! While salt gets a bad rap, a high salt diet helps to increase salt concentrations in the skin, providing increased protection from harmful microbial infections.[1]

As mentioned in Chapter 2, the potassium in kimchi may also offset the risks of high blood pressure that sometimes occurs due to high salt consumption.

It's best not to use salts that have been enriched with iodine (like many table salts), as it can affect your thyroid function. Brining and fermenting with regular table salt will make the kimchi vegetables soft and mushy. One of the qualities of good kimchi is the crunchy texture brought on by the osmolarity brining effects. Regular table salt may decrease the length of the kimchi's preservation time as well. Instead of having the kimchi last for three to five months, it may spoil after a few weeks. Mineral content is also important for healthy bacterial growth.

Finally, there are some coarse sea salts that have not had the excess bitterns (bitter byproduct of salt production) removed, which will ultimately make bitter tasting kimchi. For this reason, I recommend you buy a few and see which one makes the best tasting kimchi. For generations, my family has been using Korean solar sea salt from Sinan Bay, South Korea, because it's famous for its quality, research and manufacturing practices. It's one of the top five tidal flats in the world. What's more, it's Kosher certified and carefully made by a natural drying method in a clean ocean environment that produces highly alkaline salt. It's naturally high in essential minerals and is known for its superior taste—without bitterness. Some of this salt has been roasted at 800 degrees, making it free of pesticides, heavy metals, and radioactive waste products. But these versions do cost more.

If you're unable to find Korean solar sea salt, then coarse, white Celtic sea salt would be my second choice.

Korean Coarse Red Pepper Powder

Red pepper was introduced to kimchi making practices three hundred years ago to give kimchi a spicy, sweet and smoky pungent taste. *Capsaicin*, the active ingredient in red peppers, is what gives them functional and medicinal properties. Studies show that capsaicin promotes thermogenesis, which causes an increase in metabolism and expenditure of energy, potentially helping those with obesity.[2] Red pepper is also a good source of antioxidants, with natural compounds including flavonoids, phenolic acids, carotenoids, vitamin A, ascorbic acid (vitamin C) and tocopherols.[3] As discussed above, antioxidants help fight off the free radicals that are linked to aging and

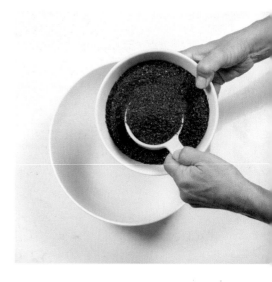

many diseases. Additionally, red pepper powder has a marked influence on the growth of LAB (lactic acid bacteria) in kimchi, such as the strain *Weissella cibaria*,[4] so if you can handle a little spice, I absolutely recommend it for maximum probiotic benefit.

The amount of red pepper powder used in each recipe depends on the degree of spiciness you want, the coarseness of the powder and the type of kimchi you're making. If too much is added while preparing the kimchi paste, you'll pick up more bitter notes. The kimchi will also take longer to ferment, which will affect the optimal growth of the kimchi microbiome. As Korean scientists discovered in 2013, red pepper serves a very important role in extending the life of the kimchi by slowing the fermentation process.[5] By adding red pepper powder, your kimchi will last longer—so don't be afraid to use it! You can make milder tasting kimchi by reducing the amount of red pepper, but know that the fermentation time will be quicker, and the kimchi will need to be eaten in a timely manner. Also, without the red pepper you may have the urge to consume way more kimchi than your gut can handle, so make sure you don't overdo it!

When buying Korean red pepper powder, look at the color and the coarseness of the flakes. The color needs to be red with a hint of dark orange. If the powder is more of an orange color, like a pumpkin, this indicates that it has been sitting on the shelf for a while and has likely oxidized. If the red pepper powder is a *really* dark red, like a maroon, it will make your kimchi dark, which will not be visibly appetizing.

Look for coarse red pepper powder that's been grown in South Korea, rather than China.

As for the coarseness of the red pepper powder, look for one where each flake size is around two millimeters in diameter. If it's been milled down to a fine powder like paprika, it'll oxidize faster and the paste consistency will be more like mud.

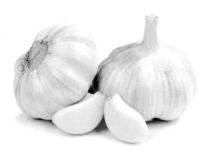

Finally, look for coarse red pepper powder that's been grown in South Korea, rather than China. Although there's a big difference in cost, you'll appreciate the level of purity in the Korean version. On the package label, look for "Product of Korea" or "Origin: Korea", rather than "P.R.O.C.", "Origin: China", "Chine" or "Product of China."

Garlic

No country on earth consumes more garlic per capita than Korea. In fact, I have never made kimchi without fresh garlic—*manuel*, as it's called. My mother says that you can make any type of kimchi, as long as you have salt and garlic.

Ginger, red pepper and pear bring more flavor to kimchi, but these are not essential ingredients the way that garlic is.

Garlic contains various medicinal compounds including allicin that are known to act as potent antioxidants.[6] It also helps with lowering LDL cholesterol[7] and has antibacterial properties.

The allicin compound found in garlic in particular has an inhibitory effect on the actions and life-cycle of strep bacteria, making it a very helpful ally for our immune system, according to Arzanlou's 2016 study.[8] Garlic has long been hailed as an immune tonic too. One study found that those who supplemented with one capsule of garlic daily suffered fewer viral infections during a four-month period and recovered more quickly than those taking a placebo.[9] Not only is garlic an all-around superfood with a long list of health benefits, it's also an important contributor in the growth of lactic acid bacteria in kimchi.

One amazing story I still hear periodically from my mother is how garlic saved her girlfriend's life during the Korean War. When my mother was around eighteen years old, she had to flee down South from Inchon with her girl-friend's family. During the harrowing journey, her friend contracted cholera, a deadly intestinal bacterial infection

Korean people love the medicinal power of garlic and add it to every dish—including, of course—kimchi!

that killed most people back in those days. Her friend was close to death when her friend's mother crushed two bulbs of fresh garlic, mixed them in with some rice porridge, and fed it to her daily for one week. Slowly, she began to improve. After a while on this garlic diet, her cholera symptoms and dysentery were completely cured. Korean people love the medicinal power of garlic and add it to every dish—including, of course—kimchi!

Ginger

Ginger is a root of the *Zingiber officinale* plant that's been used in traditional Korean and Chinese Herbal Medicine for centuries to alleviate nausea and vomiting, reduce pain, heal the digestive tract and treat the common cold. It's also known as a power-

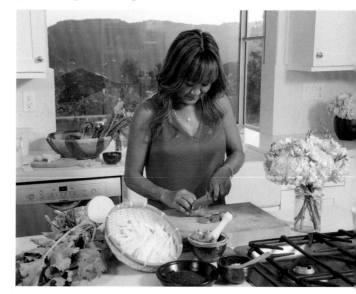

There's almost nothing that ginger can't help with.

ful decongestant and antihistamine. Now science backs up many of these claims. Gingerols, potent compounds found in ginger, have been found to help with alleviating nausea, arthritis and pain, and have anti-inflammatory, anticancer, antimicrobial and anti-allergenic properties, as well as being protective against diabetes, heart disease and liver disease.[10] There's almost nothing that ginger *can't* help with.

Not only is ginger a flavorful superstar ingredient for kimchi, it also has the amazing power to minimize the garlic smell in it. As mentioned earlier, add one-half a teaspoon of fresh ginger to hot water, or a quarter teaspoon of ginger powder to hot water, swirl it in the mouth and swallow. A few sips will remove the strong kimchi and garlic odor that some people experience.

The best way to get rid of kimchi breath is to drink a cup of ginger tea!

One more important kimchi tip. In all of my kimchi recipes, the ratio of garlic to ginger is 2:1. Use twice as much garlic as ginger.

This trick also works when washing out your dishes. To eliminate the kimchi odor from the glass jars, all you need to do is first clean the jars with soap and water, then fill them up with warm water. Add a half teaspoon of ginger powder to the clean water. Close it up with the lid on and turn it upside down for 24 hours. This way the lid can also be deodorized. You'll be amazed at how fresh it smells afterwards!

One more important kimchi tip. In all of my kimchi recipes, the ratio of garlic to ginger is 2:1. Use twice as much garlic as ginger.

Additional Ingredients

Beyond these "superstar" ingredients, kimchi can be made with a series of other tasty seasonings, spices, fruits and vegetables. Some recipes also call for:

- Organic Sweet Rice Flour
- Anchovy Fish Sauce
- Salted Shrimp Paste
- Dried Kelp (Dashima or Kombu)

The above foods don't go bad quickly, so you may wish to purchase these on your first shopping trip, along with the cucumbers, garlic, ginger, spring onions, sea salt and red pepper powder.

4 Steps to Making Kimchi

1. Brining and Preparing Vegetables

2. Preparation of Sub-ingredients

3. Mixing the Kimchi Paste and Vegetables

4. Storage and Temperature Regulation

Step One: The Art of Kimchi Cleaning and Brining

Let's start with the cleaning and brining process. All great kimchi recipes depend on first ensuring proper hygiene and the cleanliness of your equipment. Be sure to wash your hands before you begin, wipe down counters and work with very clean utensils. They don't need to be sterilized though, just nice and clean. Be sure *not* to use antibacterial soap on your hands. This type of soap kills both bad *and* good bacteria. Kimchi needs no "starter" culture, it actually gets the lactic acid bacteria directly *from your hands*. You are the starter culture!

Be sure not to use antibacterial soap on your hands. This type of soap kills both bad and good bacteria. Kimchi needs no "starter" culture, it actually gets the lactic acid bacteria directly from your hands. You are the starter culture!

The key to kimchi fermentation and optimal lactic acid bacteria growth is in the art of brining.

The standard definition of brining is "a method of soaking a food product in a saturated salt water solution." Salt is nature's disinfectant. Brining eliminates undesirable pathogenic bacteria and fungi through a process of osmotic activity, which can decrease microbial toxin development. The water is drawn out of the vegetable's cell walls as it goes from a low sodium to a high sodium environment.

The beauty of lactic acid bacteria is that it grows rapidly in a salty environment, while more pathogenic bacteria struggle to grow there. Salt also prepares and "sweats" the vegetables of excess water, so that by the end of brining process, they can bend more easily without breaking. This creates the delicious crunchy texture of kimchi.

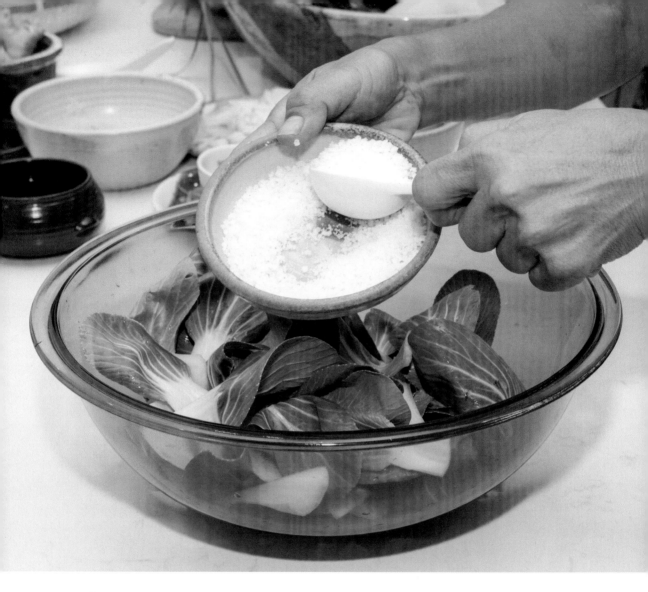

Traditionally, brining and preparation in the process of making kimchi differed in every family, just as recipes depended on the location of the family, and whether seafood and other specific sub-ingredients were available. Depending on the vegetable you're fermenting, the brining time and amount of salt used will vary, as discussed in the recipes section, Chapter 5.

As a general overview, there are three basic ways to brine vegetables for kimchi:

1. Solar Sea Salt Only

2. 10% Solar Sea Salt Solution with Water

3. Combination of Solar Sea Salt Brining
   and Sea Salt Solution

The brining technique for all of the kimchi recipes in this book is the first method, using the solar sea salt only. There are two reasons why I chose this method. First, this is the way I was taught by my mother and grandmother, and so it has the benefit of ancient wisdom on its side. Secondly, to make saline solution, you have to use tap water (unless you want to use purified water, but that would be pricey), and it can be contaminated with toxicants that are harmful to your digestive system and microbiome—including chlorine, chloramines, fluoride, arsenic, uranium and other chemicals. Better to stick with just salt!

In the recipe section, each recipe will have detailed information on how to prepare the vegetables to be brined, how much solar sea salt to use and how long to brine the vegetables for each recipe.

When brining, the first step is to wash, trim, cut and prepare the vegetables to be brined.

These vegetables are commonly used to make kimchi:

- Cucumbers
- Mustard Greens
- Baby Bok Choy
- Korean Radish
- Napa Cabbage
- Daikon
- Turnips
- Beet Tops
- Radish Tops
- Green Onion
- Purple or Green Cabbage

Second, add the prepared vegetables to a glass bowl and sprinkle the solar sea salt evenly over them. Each recipe will indicate the amount of solar sea salt to use in order to brine optimally. Put a lid on the bowl and let it sit for several hours.

If you want a more "umami" flavor to your kimchi but want to still keep it 100% vegan (fish sauce or shrimp paste gives that extra boost of seasoning), then adding kelp water to the kimchi recipe will be a great option. Best time to make kelp water is during the brining process by soak three to four pieces (3 inches x 3 inches) of dried kelp into a bowl of 4 ounces of purified water at room temperature. The kelp will slowly soften in the water, adding a mild ocean aroma and seaweed extract. This kelp water can be used as a

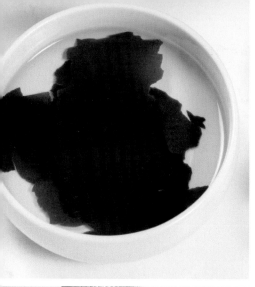

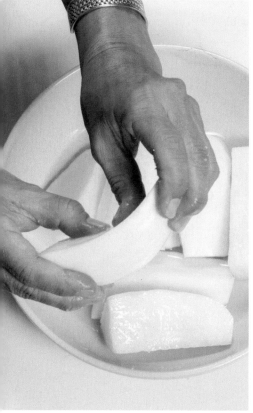

sub-ingredient instead of seafood and will add more moisture to the kimchi paste. I consider kelp water as an optional ingredient and you don't need to add it to every kimchi recipe, it tastes great even without it but I would love you to experiment with it for sure!

Third, check on the vegetables and see if they've released enough water so that they bend without snapping. More water may need to be released from the vegetables to give them that crunchy bite. If more time is needed, then distribute the vegetables and salt them a bit more on all sides. Let them "sweat" more. I believe this is the most important step, as the length of time and amount of salt used will determine if all of the pathogenic microbes have been eliminated. Checking for optimal crunchiness helps with the taste and you can create the optimal saline environment for maximum lactic acid bacteria growth.

Fourth, when the vegetables have been brined enough, rinse only *once* (for the vegan version) by dipping them into a bowl of fresh cold water quickly. If you plan on adding anchovy fish sauce or salted shrimp to your kimchi paste, you can quickly dip the vegetables twice in cool water.

Finally, drain your vegetables for 15–30 minutes in a colander. Taste it—it should taste a bit salty, but not to the point where you want to spit it out. With less water content, the vegetable should also be crunchy in texture. The brined vegetables are now ready to be mixed with the kimchi paste.

Step Two: Preparing the Sub-ingredients

So how do we make the kimchi paste? Glad you asked!

You'll wash, trim, dice, grate or julienne the kimchi sub-ingredients. Here's a list of the commonly used sub-ingredients, which will vary with each recipe:

- Garlic
- Ginger
- Garlic Chives
- Green Onions
- Onion
- Pear or Apple
- Radish

- Carrot
- Anchovy Fish Sauce
- Salted Shrimp Paste
- Dried Kelp (optional, to make kelp water)
- Sweet Rice Flour
  (optional, heated to make rice porridge)
- Sugar (optional)

I've only listed the main sub-ingredients for traditional kimchi, not the ones that are difficult to find in regular grocery stores, such as *minari* (Korean watercress—also called water dropwort).

If you're vegan, obviously you'll leave out the anchovy fish sauce and the salted shrimp paste and can replace the seafood with the kelp water as mentioned in Step 1 of the brining section, but this will change the taste and quality of the kimchi. The seafood ingredients are very salty, which helps to kill off bad bugs while adding extra flavor to the sauce. That's why I recommend rinsing the brined vegetables twice with cold water if you plan on adding the seafood ingredients. Without the seafood ingredients, you'll want to keep the brined vegetables saltier by rinsing them only once with cold water. To make 100% plant-based kimchi, you want to leave more salt on the vegetables to prevent fungal growth and eliminate pathogenic bacteria.

I personally love both types of kimchi, with and without seafood. I also love to make it exactly as my ancestors did thousands of years ago—without using any fire, gas or electricity! For that reason, I don't add sweet rice flour porridge to my kimchi paste, since a heating element is needed to make the

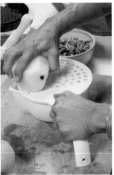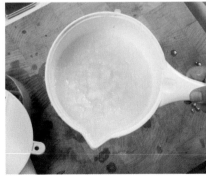

porridge. Koreans love to use the porridge because it helps with the consistency of the kimchi paste, adds volume, thickens it and makes it stick to the brined vegetables easily. Also, it's food for optimal lactic acid bacteria growth and gives the kimchi a sweeter taste. My mother uses rice porridge, but I found that grated pear is an excellent replacement and have been making kimchi without the porridge for years.

Sugar is a common ingredient added to kimchi, but kimchi studies show that the sugar is processed by the lactic acid bacteria and that you aren't really consuming it as raw, empty calories. Although the sugar and rice porridge helps the probiotics grow, I add grated fruit to bring the sweet note out in kimchi instead.

Step Three: Mixing the Kimchi Paste and Vegetables

Now that you've chopped all the sub-ingredients, add them to a glass bowl and mix thoroughly into a paste. I love this step, the alchemy of garlic, ginger and red pepper makes my mouth water and the rich red paste color is stunning! I also like to taste the kimchi paste to check on the flavor before adding it to the brined vegetables.

Depending on the type of kimchi you're making, the paste will be smeared onto the vegetables (as with Radish Kimchi), mixed into each layer (as with Napa Kimchi) or stuffed into the vegetable (as with Cucumber Kimchi). After you add the paste to your brined vegetables, you're ready to store and ferment the kimchi.

Specific detailed instructions on how to prepare the kimchi paste for each recipe can be found in the recipe section of the next chapter.

Step 4: Storage and Temperature Regulation

The final mixture of brined vegetables and kimchi paste needs to be added to storage jars that do not change the quality of the kimchi or its taste. Nor do we want to add any toxins to the kimchi. I've found that glass canning jars with lids work well, and I've accumulated many sizes and shapes over the years. Metal and plastic containers leach out residue

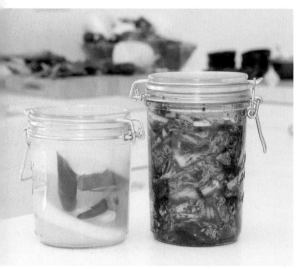

and are not recommended for kimchi storage. Some of my patients have nickel allergies, so stainless steel containers can be a big problem for them as well. I strongly recommend that you stay away from plastics. First, they present many environmental issues and second, they contain xenoestrogens, which are hormone disruptors that can leach into your food.

Using the right size jar is important. If it's too big and you don't have enough vegetables to fill up most of the jar, there will be too much oxygen in the jar and fungi growth can be a concern. If you top it off and don't leave a small amount of room for carbon dioxide gas production and fermentation, then you may have an overflow of kimchi juice after a couple of days. It's best to leave around *an inch* to *an inch-and-a-half* of room at the top of the jar. I always leave the kimchi jar in a large bowl the first few days of fermentation, just in case there is overflow.

When you pack the jar, you also want to make sure to pack the vegetables down well. Fill the jar halfway and use your fist or a wooden spoon to push the vegetables down, squeezing out as much oxygen and as many bubbles as possible. This pushes the liquid out of the vegetables, locking in the paste and juices. If the surface of the vegetable is exposed without any of the paste or juice, fungi can grow there, where oxygen is readily available. Continue this process of packing down the vegetables until the jar is full, remembering to leave about an inch at the top.

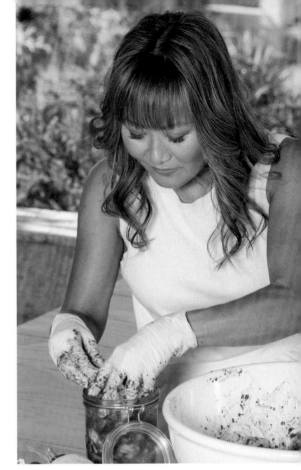

I've read online about people's kimchi jars breaking from the overexpansion of fermentation. This has never happened to me because I "burp" the jar by unscrewing the lid halfway, releasing the carbon dioxide gas after the initial 24–48 hours of fermentation. You can also buy the fancy fermentation kits with the gas releasers already built into the lids. The burping lids don't make sense for me due to my kimchi refrigerator. It's deep and wide, so it allows me to stack my bottles onto each other,

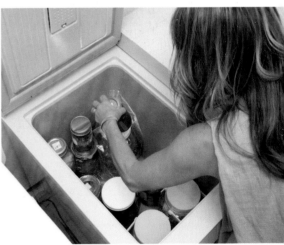

which saves space. I can have as many as thirty jars at one time!

Some people may not want the kimchi vegetables and juice touching the inside of the jar's lid. If that's a concern for you, place a sheet of parchment paper between the jar and lid. I typically don't use metal lids because over time they get rusty and will discolor the glass jar where the lid touches. I have a few old-fashion style glass jars with the wire-bale snap closure, which work well too, but they have rubber gaskets that can deteriorate over time and need replacing. I use parchment paper when I use these types of jars, as I don't like the smell of rubber mixing in with my kimchi.

Once you've packed your jars up with the vegetables, you want to *leave them out at room temperature,* away from sunlight for the initial fermentation process, before you put it into the refrigerator. Don't forget to put a bowl underneath to catch the overflow, just in case.

The initial fermentation temperature is an important element that'll govern how fast the kimchi ferments and ripens. In the summer, if the room is greater than 75 degrees Fahrenheit, I only leave the jar out at room temperature for 24–36 hours before popping it into the refrigerator, whereas in the winter, if the room is pretty cold, say below 68 degrees Fahrenheit or even colder, I may keep the jar out to ferment for two or three days. You may wish to taste the kimchi after 24 hours to see how it's coming along. The colder it is, the slower the fermentation and growth of lactic acid bacteria will be. Napa cabbage kimchi can take a long time to ferment in a cold environment and may need extra time—four to six days of initial fermentation.

This ingenious process is why Korean people were able to eat kimchi during the winter months. By adding the brined vegetables to earthenware jars and storing them underground for insulation, Koreans prevented the vegetables from freezing over, but allowed the fermentation to slowly work its magic despite the harsh weather.

A Brief Overview of Kimchi Fermentation

Lactic acid fermentation is highly desirable and a most practical method of vegetable preservation.

Once your kimchi is stored, your vegetable will undergo fermentation, in which lactic acid bacteria devour the fermentable carbohydrates in the vegetable. The lactic acid bacteria will grow, destroy bad microbes and preserve the vegetable further. As I've already mentioned, lactic acid fermentation is highly desirable and a most practical method of vegetable preservation. It's cost effective, requires no electricity or gas, minimizes wasting of fruits and vegetables and yields a highly diverse organoleptic experience—a feast for the senses!

During kimchi fermentation, the content of organic acids increases and the amount of sugar decreases. The pH decreases depending on the length of days during the initial storage at room temperature. Kimchi fermentation process is run mainly by three genera of bacteria: *Leuconostoc, Lactobacillus* and *Weisella*. The initial fermentation stage is dominated by *Leuconostoc*, followed by *Lactobacillus* and then *Weissella*, but as fermentation progresses, the growth of *Lactobacillus* and *Weissella* increase. However, after weeks of fermentation (Day 23 at 4°C), *Leuconostoc* increase in numbers again and *Lactobacillus* and *Weissella* gradually decrease.[11] In each bite of kimchi, there can be hundreds of different strains. Remember that in one tablespoon of kimchi, you can have 15 billion CFUs of LAB or more!

Remember that in one tablespoon of kimchi, you can have 15 billion CFUs of LAB or more!

> **KIMCHI FACT!**
> Korean kimchi is much less acidic (more optimal) and
> more carbonated compared to sauerkraut!

There are three phases of the kimchi lactic acid fermentation process.

At the start of Phase 1, there's a rapid drop in the pH, which increases the acidity and carbon dioxide (CO_2) levels. During this phase, lactic acid bacteria growth begins, as does the elimination of undesirable microbes. There's also a drop in natural fermentable sugars (mainly fructose and glucose), because the LAB start converting the fermentable carbohydrates into a considerable amount of mannitol. Mannitol provides a refreshing sweet taste without triggering an insulin spike, making kimchi a good food for diabetics or people suffering from other sugar imbalances. Other end products, including organic acids such as lactic acid, acetate and carbon dioxide, are produced within the first five to seven days of fermentation.

During Phase 2, there's a continuous drop in the acidity, indicated by the rapid decrease in pH and an increase in CO_2 levels. This is noticeable by the effervescent bubbles that are released as you open up a bottle of fermented kimchi. You may even feel the bubbles in your mouth as you take a bite of it, which is so titillating! LAB continues to reduce the natural sugars from around Days 7–21 of fermentation.

In the final stage of fermentation, Phase 3, there's not much of a difference in the acidity, pH or CO_2 levels, and most of the sugars have been utilized and reduced by the lactic acid bacteria. This third phase usually occurs after Day 21 and can continue for months. The preservation of kimchi depends on the salinity, the season, the storage temperature and the type of vegetable that's being fermented. For instance, cucumber kimchi is best eaten within three weeks of making it, otherwise it becomes soggy. But napa kimchi can be

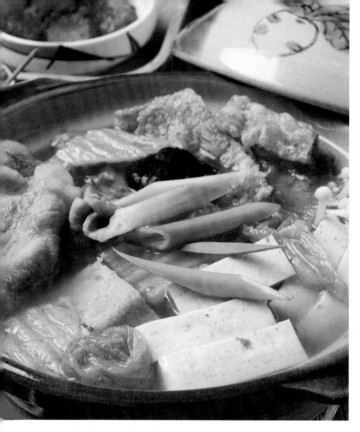

kept in the refrigerator for four to five months and still taste amazing and crunchy.

After months of storage, kimchi goes into the over-ripening stage, but don't throw it away! You can cook the over ripe napa kimchi and add it to flavor different dishes, such as kimchi fried quinoa, kimchi beef stew, kimchi pancakes, kimchi omelets and more. I use over ripe kimchi to make the traditional *kimchi jjigae*, a stew-like meal full of vegetables and *doenjang*, fermented soybean paste.

15 Kimchi Making Tips

1. Use Korean solar sea salt or white Celtic sea salt.

2. Use Korean red pepper coarse powder made in Korea, not in China.

3. Use fresh garlic and ginger, not powdered.

4. Use a glass jar that's the right size, fill it to the top, and leave 1-2 inches for carbon dioxide gas production and the release of extra water. The less oxygen the vegetables are exposed to, the better the lactic acid bacteria growth.

5. Easy on the ginger. Garlic to ginger ratio is always 2:1.

6. Vegan kimchi needs a longer time brining (fish sauce and shrimp paste add extra salt to the kimchi paste).

7. Adding sugar is optional. Sugar is actually more "food" for the growth of lactic acid bacteria, so you won't be consuming it when the kimchi is perfectly ripe. Low calorie superfood!

8. Green onions can make the kimchi juice "sticky." No need for concern, it's fine to eat but if it bothers you, use chives or garlic chives.

9. Taste the brined kimchi before mixing in the kimchi paste. It should taste salty but not to the point of wanting to spit it out.

10. Extra kimchi paste is better than not having enough. The optimal amount of kimchi sauce will affect the speed of fermentation, yeast overgrowth and taste.

11. As you are filling the jar, periodically push the content down with a spoon to release as much oxygen as possible and express more liquid out of the vegetables.

12. Put a bowl underneath the kimchi container, just in case there's overflow during the first few days of fermentation.

13. Try not to open the lid during the first few days of fermentation unless you're taste testing to see how ripe it is before refrigeration. I usually taste it after 24 hours.

14. The best temperature for the refrigerator is between 37 and 41 degrees Fahrenheit (3 to 5 degrees Celsius). Too cold will take a long time to ripen, too warm can spoil the kimchi.

15. Drink ginger tea to get rid of kimchi breath. And it's great as a digestive aid too!

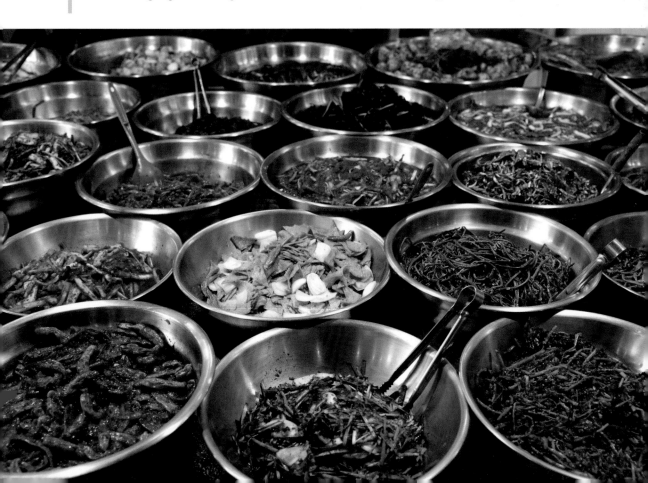

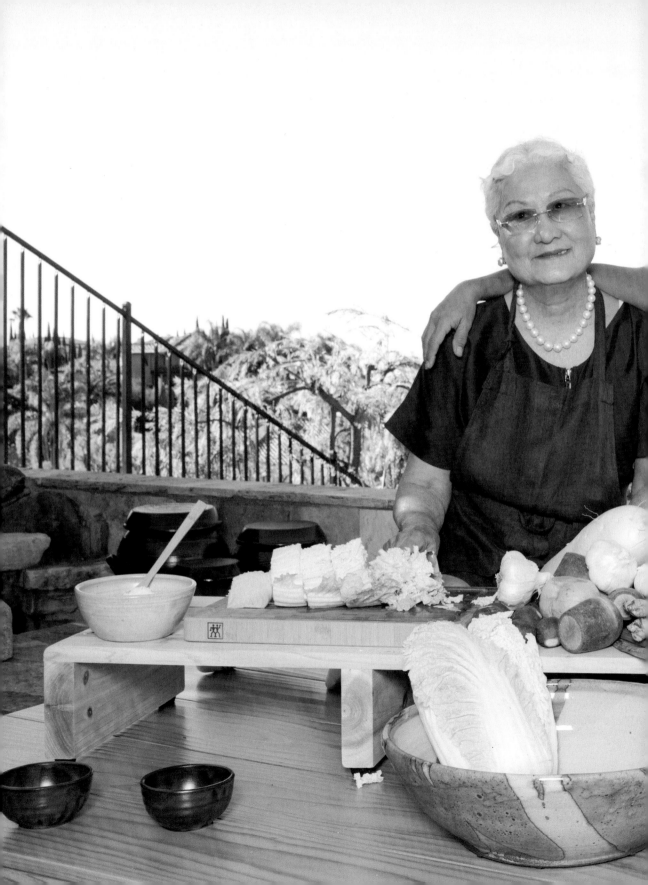

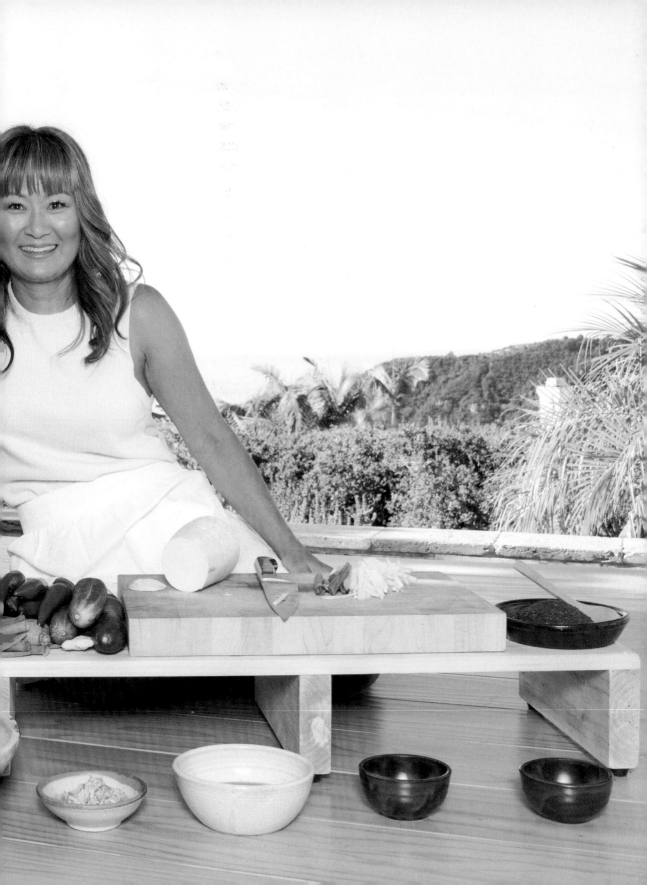

Chapter 5   *Kimchi Diet™ Recipes*

These are some of my family's absolute favorite kimchi recipes and they're listed in the order that they're to be made and eaten, according to The Kimchi Diet™ plan. They've been handed down through multiple generations, they're tried and true and I offer them to you with love. Enjoy!

Here's a Quick Summary of The Kimchi Diet™ Timeline again for your convenience.

Phase 1: Days 1–14

Day 1: Make Cucumber Kimchi.

Day 3–4: Start eating 2 to 3 pieces from one cucumber kimchi floret daily.

Day 7–8: Work up to eating the entire cucumber kimchi floret daily.

Day 8: Make baby bok choy, mustard greens, radish tops or beet tops kimchi.

Day 8–14: Continue to eat 1 cucumber kimchi floret daily.

Phase 2: Days 14–28

Day 14–21: Finish off the cucumber kimchi and start eating 1 tablespoon of the Phase 2 kimchi of your choice (baby bok choy, mustard greens, radish tops or beet tops). Work up to two tablespoons per day.

Day 21: Make root vegetable kimchi (radish, daikon, turnip, or rutabaga).

Day 21–28: Continue eating Phase 2 kimchi.

Phase 3: Days 28–42

Day 28: Continue to finish off the Phase 2 kimchi and start eating one to two tablespoons of the root vegetable kimchi (radish, daikon, turnip or rutabaga).

Day 28: Make the napa cabbage kimchi.

Day 28–42: Continue to eat 2–3 tablespoons of both Phase 2 and Phase 3 kimchi daily.

Phase 4: Days 42–56 and Beyond

Day 42: Eat one to two tablespoons of napa cabbage kimchi and watch out for symptoms.

Day 42–56: Continue eating the Phase 2 & Phase 3 kimchi, whatever's left and continue incorporating napa cabbage kimchi into your diet. Work up to eating 4 tablespoons of kimchi per day.

4 Steps to Making Kimchi

1. Brining

Wash and trim the main vegetable(s) to be salted and brined for a specific amount of time.

2. Preparation of Kimchi Paste

Wash, trim, dice, grate or julienne the sub-ingredients.

3. Make the Kimchi Paste

Prepare paste and mix it into the brined vegetables.

4. Storage and Temperature Regulation

Add the final mixture of vegetables into storage jars and store at proper temperature.

Phase 1 Recipe: Days 1–14

Cucumber (Oi) Kimchi

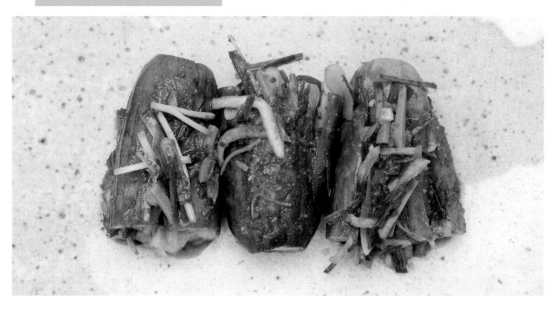

Ingredients

- 8 seedless, waxless Kirby (pickling), Persian or Lebanese cucumbers or 4 long Korean or English (hot house) cucumbers
- 2 tablespoons coarse solar sea salt

Kimchi Paste Ingredients

- 1 medium carrot, thinly sliced into matchsticks 1-1 ½ inches in length or shred with a grater if short on time

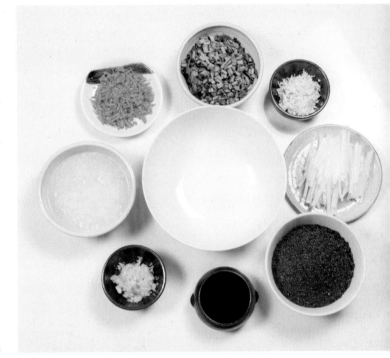

- 1 cup daikon, thinly sliced into matchsticks 1–1 ½ inches in length
- 1 cup garlic (Buchu) or common chives, chopped into ½–¾ inch pieces
- 2 teaspoons minced garlic
- 1 teaspoon grated ginger
- ½ cup grated Asian pear, Fuji apple or 2 tablespoons rice porridge* (recipe on page 145)
- 2 teaspoons anchovy fish sauce or kelp water (optional)
- ½ cup Korean red pepper powder* (reduce the amount for milder kimchi)
- 1 tablespoon purified water

*If you're sensitive to spicy foods, then red pepper powder can be omitted in all kimchi recipes, but you'll have to adjust the initial time of fermentation at room temperature by shortening a couple of hours and eat it before it over-ripens. Red pepper powder slows down the fermentation and ripening process, so you'll need to adjust accordingly. If you don't want to add red pepper or any seafood, then you'll need to make the brined vegetable a bit saltier before adding the sub-ingredient kimchi paste.

Instructions

Brining time: 1 hour

1. Wash the cucumbers and drain.

Optional: Make kelp water by soaking three to four pieces (3 inches x 3 inches) of dried kelp into a bowl of 4 ounces of purified water at room temperature.

2. Cut off the ends of each cucumber and chop them into 2–3 inch pieces. If you use Kirby's, cut them in half, or if you have longer cucumbers, cut them into 3 pieces, around 3 inches in length each.

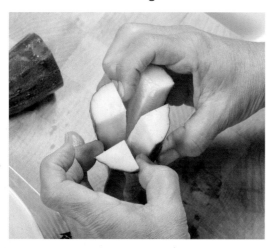

3. Place a cucumber piece on the end on the cutting board and cut them down through the diameter of the cucumber vertically (lengthwise), leaving ½ inch on the bottom of each cucumber piece uncut. Then turn 90 degree angle and perpendicularly cut through the diameter , again without cutting through completely, making an "X". This will make each 3-inch cucumber piece into a 4-petal floret, leaving room to add the kimchi paste after the brining.

4. Add the cucumber florets into a large glass or ceramic bowl and sprinkle the coarse sea salt on the inside and outside of each floret evenly. Cover the bowl and let it brine for an hour away from sunlight. After 30 minutes, you'll notice some "sweat" water in the bottom of the bowl. Toss the cucumber florets a couple of times, then let them

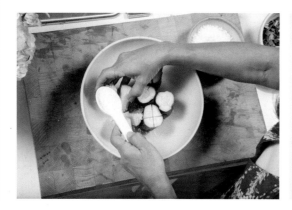
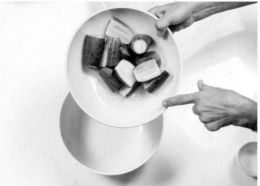

brine for the final 30 minutes. Prepare the kimchi paste ingredients by chopping, mincing and grating the sub-ingredients.

5. After brining, the cucumber should be flexible and you'll be able to bend them easily without snapping them in half. Add the brined cucumber florets to a strainer (discard the brined salty liquid) and quickly dip into a large bowl of fresh water once, to take the excess salt and any debris off. Drain in a colander for 10 minutes while you make the kimchi paste.

Kimchi Tip: If you plan on adding anchovy fish sauce to your kimchi paste, quickly dip the cucumber *twice* in the bowl of water. Try not to submerge the brined cucumber too long. Otherwise too much of the salt will be drawn out of the brined vegetables and optimal fermentation process may be affected. This "double dip" rinse applies only when you add fish sauce or shrimp paste to your recipe.

Kimchi Paste

1. In a large glass or ceramic bowl, add the garlic, ginger, grated pear, fish sauce or kelp water and red pepper flakes. Wear disposable food preparation gloves to prevent the red pepper from irritating your skin and mix the ingredients into a paste. Add the carrots, chives and daikon to the paste and mix well.

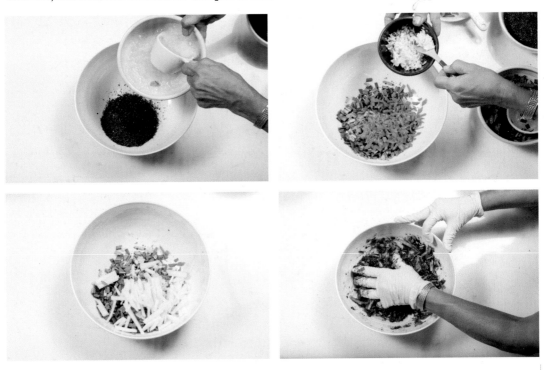

2. Stuff each cucumber floret with the chive/carrot kimchi paste. Set each stuffed floret aside in the bowl as you stuff the next floret. Don't worry if the florets break apart, it will still taste great!

3. Rub extra kimchi paste on the outside of the cucumber florets.

Kimchi Tip: It's better to have extra paste rather than not enough, make more if you have to!

Storage and Temperature Regulation

1. I like to bottle a few jars per recipe, so that while you're eating out of one jar, the others can continue their fermentation process without being disturbed. The other bottles will be untouched, bubbling with carbonation until you are ready to eat them.

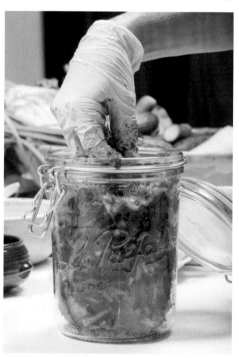

Fill the jar with the florets and when you've filled the jar half full, push the florets down with a wooden spoon to bring up the oxygen bubbles to surface. This will help prevent yeast growth. Continue to fill to the top and push as many oxygen bubbles out as possible.

Pushing down on the cucumber florets also excretes more water. This extra juice submerges the cucumber florets, which keeps the oxygen away from the vegetables and helps prevent yeast growth. Don't worry if you still see bubbles. As it ferments, more water will be released and the bubbles will come up to the surface.

Finally, add one tablespoon of purified water to any leftover kimchi paste in the bowl, and distribute evenly in each bottle before covering with a lid.

You can add parchment paper to the top of the jar and close the lid over it. If by any chance there's an overflow, the kimchi will not touch the plastic or metal lid. Parchment paper also helps keep the lid on tight.

2. Don't fill the jar completely. Leave some room at the top—about 1 inch from the top of the rim. As fermentation occurs, carbon dioxide gases produced by the LAB will build up, and more water will sweat out from the cucumbers, so the level of liquid

and kimchi will rise up to the top. If you fill the jar up all the way, there's a chance the kimchi will overflow.

Finally, put a dish or bowl under the container to catch any excess juice that may leach out during the first couple of days of fermentation. Leave the container out in room temperature (68–72 degrees Fahrenheit) away from the sun for one or two days. There is a very small possibility of cracking in your glass container. To prevent any problems, after a couple of days of fermentation, "burp" the kimchi bottle by turning the lid slowly and letting the gas out, just as you would with a bottle of carbonated water. Do this over the sink. You may be surprised by the carbon dioxide action!

3. Refrigerate between 3–5 degrees Celsius (37–41 degrees Fahrenheit) and slip a dish under to catch any possible overflow.

4. Consume as directed in Phase 1 of The Kimchi Diet™, page 97.

Note: I like to taste the fermented kimchi just before I transfer it to the refrigerator.

First, I want to see how good the kimchi tastes. I'm looking for a slightly salty, sweet, tangy and savory taste. Second, the flavor also tells me the speed of fermentation, which will govern how quickly I need to eat it before it over ripens. If I feel it needs to ferment a bit longer, I'll keep it out at room temperature for another 6–8 hours.

The speed of fermentation all depends on the amount of salt used during the brining process, as well as the temperature of the ambient environment where the jars will be stored during the initial fermentation process. In the winter, kimchi will ferment slower. In the summer months, it will ferment faster. The saltier the kimchi, the slower it ferments. And finally, if you use red pepper powder, then the kimchi will ferment slower as well. These are all nuances you'll learn as you make your kimchi from season to season.

What I love about cucumber kimchi is that it can be eaten fresh as soon as it's been prepared. This also allows anyone who's had a lot of digestive issues to introduce kimchi slowly into their diet without any strong reactions, and to gradually build up a healthier microbiome. With each day of fermentation, the LAB grows exponentially in the kimchi, and as you eat small amounts daily, you'll reap the benefits of it—and in no time you'll be transforming your inflamed, weak dysbiotic gut into one with a robust, diverse and balanced microbiome!

Cucumber kimchi is to be eaten within two weeks, but save the juice! It's still loaded with probiotics and postbiotics (LAB metabolites). You can have a couple of teaspoons a day to continue your journey towards vibrant health.

Baby Bok Choy, Mustard Greens (Gat), Radish Tops or Beet Tops Kimchi

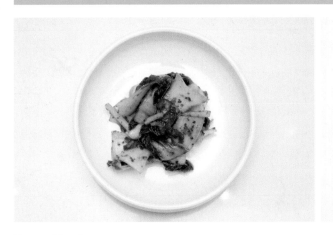 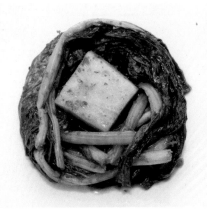

Ingredients

- 1 pound baby bok choy, mustard greens, radish or beet tops
- 1 tablespoon coarse solar sea salt

Kimchi Paste Ingredients

- 2 stalks green onion, chopped into 1-inch pieces
- ½ cup Korean radish or daikon, thinly sliced into matchsticks 1–1 ½ inches in length
- 1 teaspoon minced garlic
- ½ teaspoon grated ginger
- ¼ cup grated Asian pear, Fuji apple or 2 tablespoons rice porridge*
- 2 tablespoons Korean red pepper powder (optional)
- 1 tablespoon fish sauce or kelp water (optional)
- 1 tablespoon purified water

Instructions

Brining time: 1–2 hours

1. Soak and rinse the bok choy leaves, mustard greens, radish tops or beet tops well. Cut off the base of the stem and peel each leaf off. Drain in a colander.

2. Add the rinsed green veggies to a large glass or ceramic bowl and sprinkle the solar salt over the leaves. Add more salt to the stems and go lighter on the soft leaves to increase the "sweating," drawing out excess water from the thicker portion of the leaf.

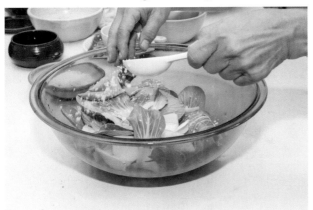 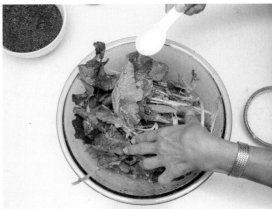

3. Cover the bowl and brine for up to 2 hours for bok choy. For mustard greens, radish and beet tops, the brining time will be shorter—around 1 hour.

4. Halfway through the brining process, turn over the leaves. You'll see there will be some water at the bottom of the bowl. Thirty minutes before the brining has finished, prepare the kimchi paste ingredients by chopping, mincing and grating the sub-ingredients.

5. By the end of the brining process, the bok choy or greens will be a bit darker in color and more flexible. Add the brined vegetables to a strainer (discard the brined salty liquid) and quickly dip the greens into a large bowl of fresh water only once to take the excess salt and any debris off. Shake off excess water and drain in a colander for 10 minutes while you prepare the kimchi paste.

Kimchi Tip: Don't forget the double dip rinse if you plan on adding fish sauce to your kimchi paste!

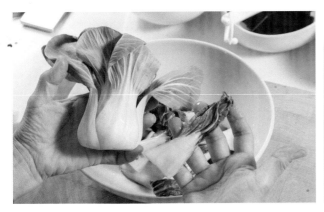 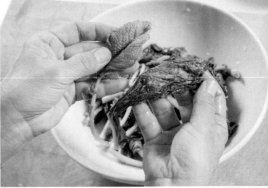

Kimchi Paste

1. In a large glass or ceramic bowl, add the garlic, ginger, grated pear, red pepper flakes and fish sauce or kelp water. Wear disposable food preparation gloves and mix the ingredients into a paste. Add the green onion and daikon to the paste and mix well.

2. Add the brined bok choy or greens and coat each leaf with the kimchi paste well.

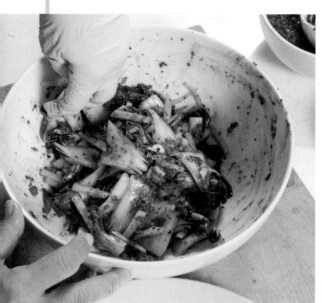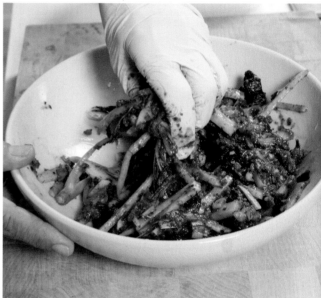

Storage and Temperature Regulation

1. Follow the same basic storage instructions as the cucumber kimchi recipe. I usually use 16 or 32-ounce glass bottles. Fill the glass container with the greens and push down on them with a wooden spoon to bring up the oxygen bubbles and squeeze out extra liquid, so it rises to the surface and submerges the greens.

2. Continue to fill to the top, pushing as many oxygen bubbles out as possible. Next, add 1 tablespoon of purified water to any leftover kimchi paste in the bowl, distributing it evenly into each bottle. Leave some space—about 1 inch from the top of the rim—before covering with a lid. You can also add parchment paper before closing the lid.

3. Leave the kimchi bottles out at room temperature (68–72 degrees Fahrenheit)—away from the sun—for 24 hours. Don't forget to add a dish under the bottle to catch any overflow of juices.

4. "Burp" each bottle after 24 hours of fermentation and taste it, as described in the Cucumber Kimchi recipe.

5. Refrigerate between 37–41 degrees Fahrenheit (3–5 degrees Celsius) and slip a dish underneath to catch any possible overflow.

6. Consume as directed in Phase 2 of The Kimchi Diet™, page 99.

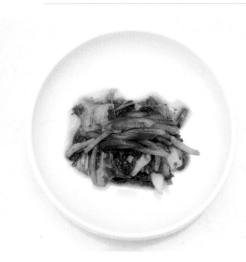

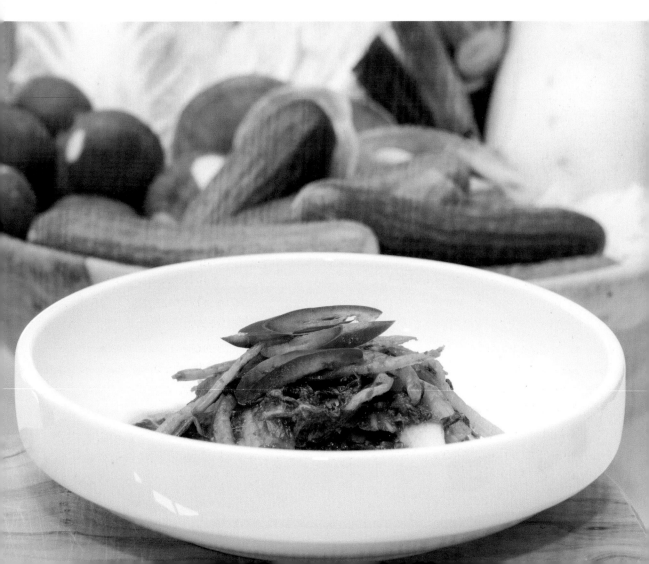

Radish (Kkakdugi) Kimchi

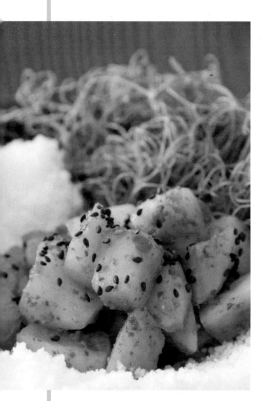

Ingredients

- 2 pounds Korean radish, daikon, turnip or rutabaga
- 2 tablespoons coarse solar sea salt

Kimchi Paste Ingredients

- 2 teaspoons minced garlic
- 1 teaspoon grated ginger
- ¼ cup garlic or common chives, chopped into ½–¾ inch pieces
- ½ cup grated Asian pear, Fuji apple or 2 tablespoons rice porridge*
- ½ cup Korean red pepper powder (use less for milder taste)
- 1 teaspoon minced salted shrimp, fish sauce or kelp water (optional)
- 1 tablespoon purified water

Instructions

Brining: 1 ½–2 hours

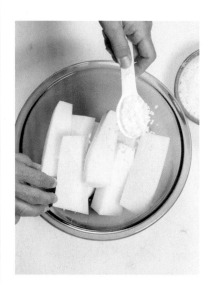

1. Rinse, scrub and cut out any areas of bruising or imbedded dirt. Use a potato peeler to peel off the skin. You can leave the peel on as long as it's clean. Cut the radish lengthwise, 1 1/2 X 4 inch pieces and add to a large glass or ceramic bowl.

Optional: Make kelp water by soaking three to four pieces (3 inches x 3 inches) of dried kelp into a bowl of 4 ounces of purified water at room temperature. Cover and set aside.

2. Sprinkle the sea salt over the cubed radish evenly. Cover and brine for 1 ½–2 hours away from sunlight.

3. Halfway through the brining process, you'll find that water has been released from the radish cubes and is sitting at the bottom of the bowl. Toss the radish cubes and let them sit for the second half of the brining time.

4. By the end of the brining process, the radish cubes will have more "give" to them. Add the brined radish to a strainer (discard the brined salty liquid) and quickly dip into a bowl of fresh water once to rinse away any excess salt or debris off. Drain in a colander for 10 minutes while you prepare the kimchi paste.

Don't forget the double dip rinse if you plan on adding fish sauce to your kimchi paste!

Kimchi Paste

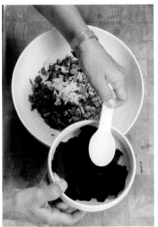 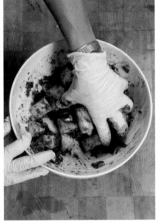

1. In a large glass or ceramic bowl, add the garlic, ginger, grated pear, red pepper flakes and minced salted shrimp, fish sauce or kelp water. Wear disposable food preparation gloves and mix the ingredients into a paste. Add the green chives to the paste and mix well.

2. Add the drained, brined radish cubes to the kimchi paste and coat the cubes with the paste evenly.

Storage and Temperature Regulation

1. Follow the same basic storage instructions as in the cucumber kimchi recipe (page 132). Fill the glass container with the brined and seasoned radish and push down with a wooden spoon to bring up the oxygen bubbles. This will squeeze out extra liquid to the surface, submerging the radish.

If you don't see any extra liquid, don't worry. During the fermentation process, more water will "sweat" out, increasing the kimchi juice volume.

2. Continue to fill to the top and push as many

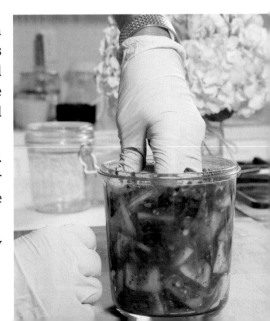

oxygen bubbles out as possible. Then add 1 tablespoon of purified water to the extra kimchi paste left in the bowl and distribute it evenly into each bottle. Leave some space—about 1 inch from the top of the rim—before covering with a lid. You can also add the parchment paper before closing the lid if you want. Place a dish underneath to catch any overflow of kimchi juice.

3. Leave the kimchi bottles at room temperature away from the sun for 2-3 days, and "burp" each bottle after a couple of days of fermentation, as described in the Cucumber Kimchi recipe. Do a taste test before refrigeration.

4. Refrigerate between 37-41 degrees Fahrenheit (3-5 degrees Celsius) and slip a dish underneath to catch any possible overflow.

5. Consume as directed in Phase 3 of The Kimchi Diet™, page 100.

Note: Radish kimchi lasts longer than most kimchi and can be kept in the refrigerator for months. The kimchi juice is absolutely delicious, especially after 4-6 weeks of fermentation. I have drizzled it over eggs, vegetables and even quinoa—spicing up my meals. I've also used the radish juice instead of spicy Tabasco sauce for my Virgin Bloody Mary drinks and it tastes amazing! You can find how to get the recipe in the Resource section on page 153.

Phase 4 Recipe: Days 42–56

Napa Cabbage (Baechu) Kimchi

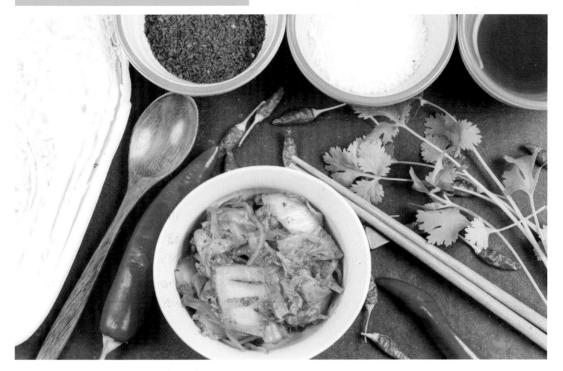

Ingredients

- 1 large Napa cabbage
- ½ cup course solar sea salt

Kimchi Paste Ingredients

- ½ cup Korean radish or daikon, thinly sliced into matchsticks 1–1 ½ inches in length
- 2 teaspoons minced garlic
- 1 teaspoon grated ginger
- ¼ cup garlic or common chives, chopped into ½–¾ inch pieces
- ½ cup grated Asian pear, Fuji apple or 2 tablespoons rice porridge*
- ½ cup Korean red pepper powder
- 2 teaspoons anchovy fish sauce, shrimp paste or kelp water (optional)
- 2 tablespoons purified water

Instructions

Brining Time: 4 hours

1. Cut the cabbage in half lengthwise. Then cut it again, so that you have four quartered cabbage pieces. The stem should be attached and will hold all the leaves in place. Peel off and discard all wilted or damaged leaves and rinse the rest thoroughly under cold running water, especially around the stem. There will be a slippery feel to the stem at first, but as you run your thumb several times over it, you will notice a "sak sak" clean sound under the running water. Wash all four cabbage pieces well and turn them upside down in a colander to drain.

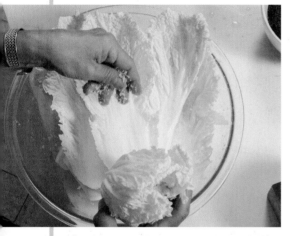

2. Place one drained cabbage quarter to a large glass or ceramic bowl, facing up so the leaves are exposed. Starting from the bottom leaf up, sprinkle the course sea salt evenly throughout each leaf, spreading more salt on the thicker portion of each leaf, closer to the stem, Use up to ½ cup of sea salt for the entire napa cabbage.

3. Collapse the leaves tightly together and leave in a large glass or ceramic bowl with the inside of the cabbage facing up, to keep the salt tightly bound inside the cabbage leaves. Add a heavy dish on top of the cabbage to keep the leaves closed. Cover and leave at room temperature away from the sun for 4 hours.

4. A couple of hours into the brining process, check on the cabbage. The stem will look shinier, the leaves brighter in color and noticeably smaller in size due to the "sweating" caused by the salt pulling the water content out of the leaves. The leaves will be flexible enough for the stem to bend without breaking. This will create a great texture and crunchiness in the kimchi. You'll see extra water at the bottom of the bowl—don't throw it out. Turn the cabbage over and leave it alone for another couple of hours. Again, this depends on how salty you want your kimchi.

Optional: Make kelp water by soaking three to four pieces (3 inches x 3 inches) of dried kelp into a bowl of 4 ounces of purified water at room temperature. Cover and set aside.

Thirty minutes before the brining has finished, prepare the kimchi paste ingredients by chopping, mincing and grating the sub-ingredients.

5. Add the brined cabbage to a strainer (discard the brined salty liquid) and quickly dip into a bowl of fresh cold water once to rinse away any excess salt or debris. This is the point I like to taste the brined Napa cabbage. It should be crunchy in texture and salty like the ocean. If it's too salty, then you can rinse it one more time.

Kimchi Tip: Don't forget the double dip rinse if you plan on adding fish sauce to your kimchi paste!

6. Gently squeeze the water out and let it drain in a colander for 15 minutes while you're preparing the kimchi paste.

Kimchi Paste

1. In a large glass or ceramic bowl, add the garlic, ginger, grated pear, red pepper flakes and anchovy fish sauce, shrimp paste or kelp water. Wear disposable food preparation gloves and mix the ingredients into a paste. Add the green chives and daikon to the paste and mix well.

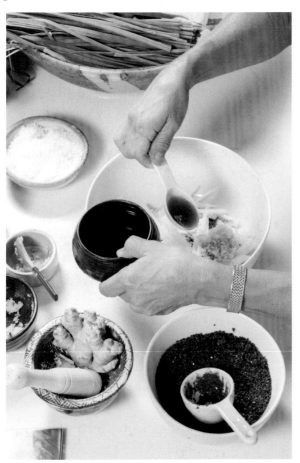

2. Peel off one large outside brined leaf from each half of the cabbage and set aside to be used during the storage step.

3. Before adding the kimchi paste to the brined cabbage, you have a choice to either cut up the cabbage into bite size pieces and then add the kimchi paste, which will make it easier for you to eat after fermentation—or you can add the kimchi paste to the cabbage with the leaves attached to the stem, letting it ferment and then cutting it up each time you want to eat some.

I personally love to make it both ways, but traditionally Korean people believe it's more honorable and aesthetically beautiful to cut up the kimchi as it's about to be served to their guests.

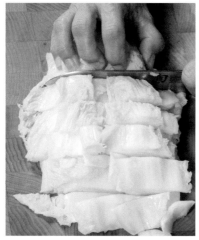

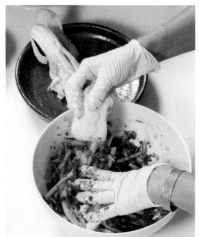

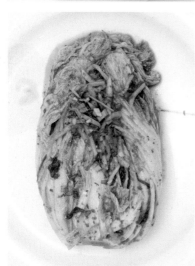

4. I'll give you both versions here:

Speedy version (Mak Kimchi)

Cut up the brined cabbage into small, bite-sized 1–2 square inch pieces and add it to the large glass bowl of kimchi paste. While wearing disposable food preparation gloves, mix the kimchi paste into the brined cabbage well. It's now ready to be added to the glass containers.

Traditional version (Baechu Kimchi)

Wear disposable food preparation gloves and add the quartered brined cabbage to the large bowl of kimchi paste. With the inside of the leaves facing up, peel back all of the leaves down to the last layer and smear the paste onto each leaf.

Add more towards the stem of each leaf, where it needs heavier seasoning. Do this to each leaf layer.

Once all layers have been seasoned, tightly wrap the outer layers of leaves around the inner leaves, keeping the paste inside. Gently set aside so it doesn't unravel and repeat with the rest of the brined cabbage. You should have enough kimchi paste to season each of the quartered brined cabbage pieces. It's now ready to be added to the glass containers.

Storage and Temperature Regulation

1. Use two 16-ounce bottles or one 32-ounce bottle to make kimchi from one whole Napa cabbage.

2. For both versions, follow the same basic storage instructions as the Cucumber Kimchi recipe. Fill the glass container with the seasoned Napa cabbage and push down with a wooden spoon to bring up the oxygen bubbles. This will squeeze out extra liquid to the surface, submerging the cabbage pieces.

For the traditional version, you can add all four wrapped cabbage pieces into a 32-ounce bottle.

It's more difficult to get the gas bubbles out of the traditional version without breaking apart the ball of cabbage.

3. Add 2 tablespoons of purified water to any extra kimchi paste that's left in the bowl and distribute it evenly into the bottle(s).

4. Leave about 1 inch of space from the top of the rim. Before closing up the lid, add a single layer of the brined cabbage to the top of the seasoned cabbage. This is the one that was set aside in Step 2 of the Kimchi Paste section. This will look like a "toupee" on top of the seasoned cabbage, and will prevent the oxygen from coming into contact with the seasoned cabbage during the fermentation process, reducing yeast growth.

5. You can also add the parchment paper before closing the lid if you choose to. Add a dish underneath the bottles to catch any overflow of kimchi juice. Leave the kimchi bottles at room temperature away from the sun for 2 days and "burp" each bottle every day. Do a taste test before refrigeration.

6. Refrigerate between 37–41 degrees Fahrenheit (3–5 degrees Celsius) and slip a dish under to catch any possible overflow.

7. Consume as directed in Phase 4 of The Kimchi Diet™, page 100.

*Rice Porridge Recipe

Ingredients

- 2 tablespoons organic sweet rice flour
- 1 cup purified water

In a small pot, add 1 cup of purified water and 2 tablespoons of organic sweet rice flour. Stir continuously and bring to boil. It will thicken into a porridge. Transfer the rice porridge into a bowl and set aside to cool down while preparing the kimchi ingredients and paste.

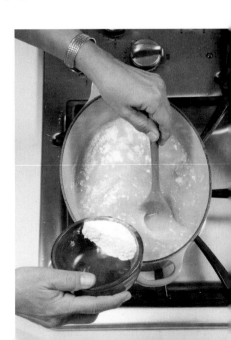

Final Note

Kimchi has finally begun to get its deserved status on the global stage of foods. This simple fermented food that my ancestors ate because they needed to preserve scarce vegetables over the winter is now popping up in food trucks, trendy restaurants and health food stores the world over. Personally, I couldn't be happier that kimchi's reputation as a superfood has spread beyond Korea to all corners of the world. I truly hope to be one of the world's leading ambassadors of the kimchi revolution: a global food for the health and protection of future generations.

I think kimchi is great not only for the health reasons I've outlined in this book, but also because it represents something simple and ancient that our modern world often forgets: tradition. The history of kimchi is filled with hands chopping vegetables as the dark days of winter began, with stories that mothers told their daughters, and with the feeling of siwonhan-mat—optimal physical contentment—that families shared during a great meal. Kimchi is not something that requires first-world money or technology to make. It's a superfood that no lab and no scientist can hope to duplicate. I imagine kimchi as part of a global food culture that the poorest people in the world as well as those who are more fortunate can embrace equally. For the price of a little garlic, ginger, salt and any local vegetable, this wonder food can belong to anyone!

I foresee kimchi as a symbol of our global era. It's decidedly ancient—stored in pots under the earth by pre-industrial peoples—and thoroughly modern, as it spreads into supermarkets and crosses cultural and linguistic traditions. Kimchi is a unifier across culture, since it offers the human body some of the most elemental and rejuvenating nutrition available.

I'm honored that you've decided to undertake the journey of The Kimchi Diet™ with me, and I'm certain that within just a few weeks, you'll see just how magical it can be. I know that if you keep up the program, make kimchi week after week and integrate its histories, tales and tastes into your home, you'll have a whole new outlook on your health—and perhaps even your life!

To your vibrant health,

Dr. Susanne

Acknowledgements

Writing this book has truly been a labor of love for me. My passion for kimchi goes all the way back to my childhood roots in Korea, and I've poured all of that love—along with heaps of cutting edge science to back up kimchi health claims—into this book. I know that I couldn't have done it without all of the encouragement, support, guidance and inspiration that I've received from my family, friends, mentors, colleagues, and so many others along the way.

First, I'm eternally grateful to my beloved mother, Suh Jung Hee and maternal grandmother, Oh Myong Kun for sharing their incredibly tasty kimchi recipes and ancient kimchi secrets with me, having been passed down from previous generations of women in our family. My love for you is endless.Thank you so much for instilling in me a deep fondness and recognition of all that kimchi has to offer us and for teaching me how to create a simple, traditional food that's not only forever changed my life and the future health of my family, but will now go on to impact so many other lives around the world with the release of this book. You are spreading your love far and wide! To my late father, John Hanjin Chun, I miss you Dad. I always think of you when I eat rice mixed with gochujang (fermented red pepper paste) and kimchi—your favorite! You would have been so proud of this book!

My son Cody and my husband George are my lifeline and have done so much to support my journey in completing this book. Cody has always said that he feels more Korean than Russian (his father's ancestry), and it was his idea for us as a family to visit Korea during the summer of 2013 before heading off for college. That trip was my first time back to Korea since I'd left in 1975 at 12 years old—and it was there that my love affair with kimchi really began, and my desire to share it with the world. George has always been my biggest fan, and I'm so lucky to have his ever-present love, encouragement and belief in me. I love you both forever, so deeply.

Many thanks also to my awesome siblings, Lisa Rodondi, Charles Chun and Maggie Drake—whom I love and cherish—for their encouragement and excitement about this book and the thousands of Korean meals we have had together as a family—always with kimchi on the side! And to my cousins, Hanna and Arnie DeLuca, thank you so much for your enthusiasm and energy toward everything I do, you are both so appreciated and loved!

All of my amazing circle of friends have contributed in one way or another to the creation of this book and I thank each of you from the bottom of my heart. But I want to call out a few here, starting with Rose Pinard—my best friend since 4 years old—and my kimchi sister. Rose and I love to go to Korean restaurants and eat our share of kimchi together (LYLAS Rose)! And Christiane Burchard for her treasured friendship—and for being my favorite travel buddy! I'm forever grateful to my beautiful, brilliant girlfriends Dr. Hyla Cass, Dr. Joan Rosenberg, Dr. Nalini Chilkov, Lavinia Errico and Grace Suh. Your ongoing love and support gave me the courage and inspiration to share my knowledge and passions with the world. Love you all so much! To my accountability buddy, Chris Maskill, I love the way you make me do the real work! So grateful for your honest opinion and encouragement!

I certainly wouldn't be where I am today without my world-class mentors, starting with JJ Virgin—my buddy for over 30 years and a mentor of mine for many years in building my nutrition practice and online business. It was JJ who introduced me to Brendon Burchard, who became another cherished mentor of mine. Brendon inspired me to not only keep going at 50 years old when I was planning to retire, but also inspired me to start working in a much bigger way, so that I could begin to serve a much wider audience than I ever could in my clinical practice. I owe much of my creative drive and my ability to do this work to Brendon and I am forever grateful. To Chad Johnson of Strategic Coach, thank you so much for your enthusiasm and support! I have learned so much from you these past two years. You have been instrumental to my focus and mental clarity, I am finally getting out of my own way! Thank you Michael Fishman of Consumer Health Summit—I cherish all that I have learned from you and look forward to many more years to come!

Big thanks to all of the teachers, chiropractors, functional medicine health practitioners, allergy experts, doctors and colleagues that I've met over the years in various seminars, expert groups and at health conferences (Institute of Functional Medicine, ACAM, AAEM, A4M, IHS, Strategic Coach, Consumer Health Summit, Mindshare, Santa Monica Functional Medicine Group, and so much more!) I appreciate you all so much for the inspiration, education, collaborations and giving me the opportunity to pick your brain!

To Cynthia Pasquella, JJ Virgin and my Unicorn Club sisters, I appreciate every one of you for your friendship and encouragement! You are all so amazingly brilliant and beautiful, from the inside out!

Many thanks to my patients, students and health community, whom I serve daily at my clinical practice and through the Wellness for Life radio show, my blog, social media, and my books. You all keep me motivated and engaged to learn more and do more—always. I want you to live your best life today!

Special thanks to Dr.Tom O'Bryan for writing the foreword for this book. Tom is a long-time colleague and his knowledge and appreciation of gut health make him the perfect fit for contributing his thoughts on this important topic!

Kudos to Kelli MacTaggart of MacTaggart Media for capturing the magic of kimchi photographs and to my stepson, Cory Gomberg of Poseidon Studios who stylized this stunning book cover.

Forever grateful to everyone on the Kimchi book production team for your amazing dedication and work ethic: Zen Dochterman, Meghann Milton, Cosmin Augustin Silaghi, Petre Nicolescu, Vobiscum Printing, Kathy Hadzibajric, Amy Thomas, Frank Mercado, Hannah Diffenderffer and Duke Gallo. This book is only here because of each of you. Thank you so much!

I want to thank Na Mi Nah and WIKIM (World Institute of Kimchi), Kimchi Master Chef Lee Ha Yeon, Dr. Jia Choi, CEO of O'ngo Food Communications, Simon Cho and Organic Red Pepper manufacturer Kang Kyu Heon of Anmyundo Nonghyup and EZ, my Korean Interpreter and videographer. I so appreciate you for making my self-funded 2018 research trip to Korea such a success and one of the best experiences of my life.

And Finally, I can't leave out my gratitude for the people of Korea as a whole—and their profound appreciation and enjoyment of kimchi—which has brought Korea to a much healthier state of well-being than it would be without this magical healing food! Now I hope to sprinkle a little bit of this magic all around the world!

Resources

There's so much more information I would like to share with you about living the kimchi life but could not be included in this book, so I have added all of my resources to one place. I have mentioned in this book including what to look for when you buy kimchi ingredients, the videos of my recent trip to Korea, exotic kimchi recipes, PDF download of the Ultimate Wellness For Life Food List/Anti-Inflammatory Nutrition Plan, and much more! You can grab all of my complimentary resources here:

Drsusanne.com/kimchiresources

Join in on the kimchi revolution and be a part of the Kimchi Diet facebook group! Check out the kimchi recipes, articles, videos and Q & A. Our health conscious community is a place where everyone can ask each other questions and post their own kimchi recipes, photos and videos too! I want your to share your "wins" and sprinkle a little of your kimchi magic!

Drsusanne.com/kimchidietgroup

Private Practice

For person to person, Skype, Facetime, or phone consultations:
Dr. Susanne Bennett
1526 14th Street, Suite 111
Santa Monica, CA 90404
Tel: 310-315-1514
Fax: 310-315-1504
Email: help@drsusanne.com

Dr. Susanne's Websites

thekimchidiet.com
kimchidetox.com
drsusanne.com
mightymito.com
the7dayallergymakeover.com
purigenex.com

Dr. Susanne's Wellness For Life Radio

wellnessforliferadio.com

 Kimchi Diet Facebook Group: drsusanne.com/kimchidietgroup

 facebook.com/drsusannebennettallergyspecialist

 @drsusanne

 Dr. Susanne Bennett

Notes

1. Baquero, F. & Nombela, C. (2012). *The microbiome as a human organ. Clinical microbiology and infection: the official publication of the European Society of Clinical Microbiology and Infectious Diseases, (4): 2-4.*

2. Sampson, Timothy R. & Mazmanian, Sarkis K. (2015). Control of Brain Development, Function, and Behavior by the Microbiome. *Cell Host Microbe, 17(5):565-76.*

3. Lerner, A., Neidhöfer, S. & Matthias, T. (2017). The Gut Microbiome Feelings of the Brain: A Perspective for Non-Microbiologists. *Microorganisms, 5(4).*

4. Cenit, M.C., Nuevo, I.C., Codoñer-Franch, P., Dinan, T.G. & Sanz, Y. (2017). Gut microbiota and attention deficit hyperactivity disorder: new perspectives for a challenging condition. *European Society of Child and Adolescent Psychiatry, (9):1081-1092.*

5. Cenit, M.C., Nuevo, I.C., Codoñer-Franch, P., Dinan, T.G. & Sanz, Y (2017). Gut microbiota and attention deficit hyperactivity disorder: new perspectives for a challenging condition. *Frontiers in cellular neuroscience, 9:392.*

6. Friedland, R.P. (2015). Mechanisms of molecular mimicry involving the microbiota in neurodegeneration. *Journal of Alzheimer's disease: JAD, 45(2):349-62.*

7. Dzutsev, A., Goldszmid, R.S., Viaud, S., Zitvogel, L. & Trinchieri, G. (2015). The role of the microbiota in inflammation, carcinogenesis, and cancer therapy. *European journal of immunology, 45(1):17-31.*

8. Cenit, M.C., Sanz, Y. & Codoñer-Franch, P. (2017). Influence of gut microbiota on neuropsychiatric disorders. *World journal of gastroenterology, 23(30):5486-5498.*

9. Guernier et al. (2017). Gut microbiota disturbance during helminth infection: can it affect cognition and behaviour of children? *BMC infectious diseases, 17(1):58.*

10. David et al. (2014). Diet rapidly and reproducibly alters the human gut microbiome. *Nature, 505(7484):559-63.*

11. Lynch, D.B., Jeffery I.B. & O'Toole, P.W. (2015). *The role of the microbiota in ageing: current state and perspectives.*

12. Senthong et al. (2016). Intestinal Microbiota-Generated Metabolite Trimethylamine-N-Oxide and 5-Year Mortality Risk in Stable Coronary Artery Disease: The Contributory Role of Intestinal Microbiota in a COURAGE-Like Patient Cohort. *Journal of the American Heart Association, 5(6).*

13. Tang et al. (2015). Gut microbiota-dependent trimethylamine N-oxide (TMAO) pathway contributes to both development of renal insufficiency and mortality risk in chronic kidney disease. *Circulation research, 116(3):448-55.*

14. Everard et al. (2013). Cross-talk between Akkermansia muciniphila and intestinal epithelium controls diet-induced obesity. *Proceedings of the National Academy of Sciences of the United States of America, 110(22):9066-71.*

Introduction

1. Mark Maginer. (2003, June 17) In an age of SARS, Koreans tout kimchi cure. *Los Angeles Times.*

2. Korea Herald. (2010, March 30). Scientists show kimchi may help combat AI, SARS. *Korea Herald.*

3. World Institute of Kimchi (2018, July 26) Kimchi, a well-known traditional fermented Korean food, has proven effective against influenza virus. *PR Newswire.*

4. Bonaz, B., Bazin, T., & Pellissier, S. (2018). The vagus nerve at the interface of the microbiota-gut-brain axis. *Frontiers in Neuroscience, 12, 1-8*

5. Shreiner, A. B., Kao, J. Y., & Young, V. B. (2015). The gut microbiome in health and in disease. *Current Opinion in Gastroenterology, 31(1), 69–75.*

6. Bonaz, B., Bazin, T., & Pellissier, S. (2018). The vagus nerve at the interface of the microbiota-gut-brain axis. *Frontiers in Neuroscience, 12, 1-8.*

Chapter 1: History of Kimchi

1. UNESCO (2013). Kimjang, making and sharing kimchi in the Republic of Korea.

2. Hongu, N., Kim, A. S., Suzuki, A., Wilson, H., Tsui, K.C., & Park, S. (2017). Korean kimchi: promoting healthy meals through cultural tradition. *Journal of Ethnic Foods 4(3),* 172-180.

3. *Jakarta Post* (2017, October 6). Half of kimchi served at Korean restaurants from China: Institute. Jakarta Post.

4. World Institute of Kimchi (2015). *The Science and Culture of Kimchi: Journey into Healthy Kimchi.* Seoul: World Institute of Kimchi.

5. Park, K. & Ju, J. (2018). Kimchi and its health benefits. In K. Park, D. Kwon, K. Lee, and S. Park (Eds.). *Korean Functional Foods: Composition, Processing, and Health Benefits.* Boca Raton: CRC Press.

Chapter 2: Kimchi Science & Health Benefits

1. SELF Nutrition Data (n.d.). Napa cabbage kimchi nutrition data & calories.

2. Harvard Health Publishing (2016 October). Can gut bacteria improve your health?. *Harvard Medical School.*

3. Zhang, Y.-J., Li, S., Gan, R.-Y., Zhou, T., Xu, D.-P., & Li, H.B. (2015). Impacts of gut bacteria on human health and diseases. *International Journal of Molecular Sciences, 16(4),* 7493–7519.

4. Zhang, Y.-J., Li, S., Gan, R.-Y., Zhou, T., Xu, D.-P., & Li, H.-B. (2015). Impacts of gut bacteria on human health and diseases. *International Journal of Molecular Sciences, 16(4),* 7493–7519.

5. Worland, J. (2017 March 28). Why researchers are concerned this pesticide may cause cancer. *Time.*

6. Ren, F., Reilly, K., Kerry, J., Gaffney, M., Hossain, M. & Rai, D. (2017). Higher antioxidant activity, total flavonols, and specific quercetin glucosides in two different onion (Allium cepa l.) varieties grown under organic production: Results from a 6-Year field study. *Journal of Agricultural and Food Chemistry, 65* (25), 5122-5132.

7. Lobo, V., Patil, A., Phatak, A., & Chandra, N. (2010). Free radicals, antioxidants and functional foods: Impact on human health. *Pharmacognosy Reviews,* 4(8), 118–126.

8. Jung,S., So, B., Shin, S.; Noh, S., Jung, E., & Chae, S. (2014). Physiochemical and quality characteristics of young radish (yulmoo) kimchi cultivated by organic farming. Journal of the *Korean Food Society and Nutrition, 43(8),* 1197-1206.

9. Kwon, H., Son, K., Kim, T., Hong, S., Cho, N. (2014). Change of pesticide residues in field-sprayed young Chinese cabbages and young radishes during kimchi preparation and storage in kimchi fridge. *The Korean Journal of Pesticide Science. 18(4),* 221-227.

10. Chang, J., Kim, I., & Chang, H. (2014). Effect of solar salt on kimchi fermentation during long-term storage. *Journal of the Korean Food Society and Nutrition, 46(4),* 456-464.

11. Chang, J., Kim, I., Chang, H. (2014). Effect of Solar Salt on Kimchi Fermentation during Long-term Storage. *Journal of the Korean Food Society and Nutrition, 46(4),* 456-464.

12. Jung, J., Lee, S., Kim, J., Park, M., Bae, J., Hahn, Y., Madsen, E. & Jeon, C. (2011). Metagenomic analysis of kimchi, a traditional Korean fermented food. *Applied and Environmental. Microbiology,* 77(7), 2264-2274.

13. Robertson, R. (2017 June 14). 9 ways lactobacillus acidophilus can benefit your health. *Healthline.*

14. Santaolalla, R., Fukata, M., & Abreu, M. T. (2011). Innate immunity in the small intestine. *Current Opinion in Gastroenterology, 27(2),* 125–131.

15. Liu, R., Kim, A.H., Kwak, M.K., & Kang, S.O. (2017). Proline-based cyclic dipeptides from Korean fermented vegetable kimchi and from Leuconostoc mesenteroides LBP-K06 have activities against multidrug-resistant bacteria. *Frontiers in Microbiology, 8,* 1-15.

16. Broussard, J. & Devkota, S. (2016). The changing microbial landscape of Western society: Diet, dwellings and discordance. *Molecular Metabolism 5,* 737-742.

17. Broussard, J. & Devkota, S. (2016). The changing microbial landscape of Western society: Diet, dwellings and discordance. *Molecular Metabolism 5*, 737-742.

18. Dukowicz, A. C., Lacy, B. E., & Levine, G. M. (2007). Small intestinal bacterial overgrowth: A comprehensive review. *Gastroenterology & Hepatology, 3(2)*, 112–122.

19. Weinstock, L.B., & Walters, A.S. (2011). Restless legs syndrome is associated with irritable bowel syndrome and small intestinal bacterial overgrowth. *Sleep Medicine, 12(6)*, 610-613.

20. Erdogan, A. & Rao, S.S. (2015). Small intestinal fungal overgrowth. *Current Gastroenterology Reports, 17(16)*.

21. Ojetti, V., Pitocco, D., Scarpellini, E., Zaccardi, F., Scaldaferri, F., Gigante, G., Gasbarrini, G., Ghirlanda, G., & Gasbarrini, A. (2009). Small bowel bacterial overgrowth and type 1 diabetes. *European Review for Medical and Pharmacological Sciences, 13(6)*, 419-423.

22. Zhang, Y., Liu, G., Duan, Y., Han, X., Dong, H., & Geng, J. (2016). Prevalence of small intestinal bacterial overgrowth in multiple sclerosis: A case-control study from China. *Journal of Neuroimmunology, 301*, 83-87.

23. Center for Disease Control (2017). Antibiotic/Antimicrobial resistance.

24. Kim M. J., Kwon M. J., Song Y. O., Lee E. K., Yoon H. J., & Song Y. S. (1997). The effects of kimchi on hematological and immunological parameters *in vivo* and *in vitro*. *Journal of the Korean Society of Food Science and Nutrition, 26*, 1208–1214.

25. Kim, H., Oh, S.Y., Kang, M.H., Kim, K.N., Kim, Y., & Chang, N. (2014). Association between kimchi intake and asthma in Korean adults: the fourth and fifth Korea National Health and Nutrition Examination Survey (2007-2011). *Journal of Medicinal Food, 17(1)*, 172-178.

26. Kwon, Y.S., Park, Y.K., Chang, H.J., & Ju, S.Y. (2016). Relationship between plant food (fruits, vegetables, and kimchi) consumption and the prevalence of rhinitis among Korean adults: Based on the 2011 and 2012 Korea National Health and Nutrition Examination Survey data. *Journal of Medicinal Food, 19(12)*,1130-1140.

27. Rho, M.K., Kim, Y.E., Rho, H.I., Kim, T.R., Kim, Y.B., Sung, W.K., Kim, T.W., Kim, D.O., & Kang, H. (2017). Enterococcus faecium FC-K derived from kimchi is a probiotic strain that shows anti-allergic activity. *Journal of Microbiology and Technology, 27(6)*, 1071-1077.

28. Jeong, J.W., Choi, I.W., Jo, G.H., Kim, G.Y., Kim, J., Suh, H., Ryu, C.H., Kim, W.J., Park, K.Y., & Choi, Y.H. (2015). Anti-inflammatory effects of 3-(4'-hydroxyl-3',5'-dimethoxyphenyl) propionic acid, an active component of Korean cabbage kimchi, in lipopolysaccharide-stimulated bv2 microglia. *Journal of Medicinal Food, 18(6)*, 677-84.

29. Yang, Y., & Jobin, C. (2014). Microbial imbalance and intestinal pathologies: Connections and contributions. *Disease Models & Mechanisms, 7(10)*, 1131–1142.

30. Hakansson, A., & Molin, G. (2011). Gut microbiota and inflammation. *Nutrients, 3(6)*, 637–682.

31. Park, K. and Ju, J. (2018). Kimchi and its health benefits. In K. Park, D. Kwon, K. Lee, and S. Park (Eds.). *Korean Functional Foods: Composition, Processing, and Health Benefits.* 43-77. Boca Raton: CRC Press.

32. Woo, M., Kim, M.J., & Song, Y.O. (2018). Bioactive compounds in kimchi improve the cognitive and memory functions impaired by amyloid beta. *Nutrients, 10(10),*

33. Kim, S., Woo, M., Kim, M., Noh, J.S., & Song, Y.O. (2018). Neuroprotective effects of the methanol extract of kimchi, a Korean fermented vegetable food, mediated via suppression of endoplasmic reticulum stress and caspase cascade pathways in high-cholesterol diet-fed mice. *Journal of Medicinal Food, 21(5)* 489-495.

34. Matt, S.M., Allen, J.M., Lawson, M.A., Mailing, L.J., Woods, J.A., & Johnson, R.W. (2018). Butyrate and dietary soluble fiber improve neuroinflammation associated with aging in mice. *Frontiers in Immunology, 9.*

35. Bourassa, M.W., Alim, I., Bultman, S.J., & Ratan, R.R. (2016). Butyrate, neuroepigenetics and the gut microbiome: Can a high fiber diet improve brain health? *Neuroscience Letters, 625,* 55-63.

36. Chang, J.H., Shim, Y.Y., Cha, S.K., & Chee, K.M. (2010). Probiotic characteristics of lactic acid bacteria isolated from kimchi. *Journal of Applied Microbiology, 109(1),* 220-30.

37. Park, K. and Ju, J. (2018). Kimchi and its health benefits. In K. Park, D. Kwon, K. Lee, and S. Park (Eds.). *Korean Functional Foods: Composition, Processing, and Health Benefits* (p. 57). Boca Raton: CRC Press.

38. Marco, M., Dustin, H., Binda, S., Cifelli, C., Cotter, P., Foligne, B., Ganzle, M., Kort, R., Pasin, G., Pihlanto, A., Smid, E., Hutkins, R. (2017) Health benefits of fermented foods: Microbiota and beyond. *Current Opinion in Biotechnology 44,* 94-102.

39. Tremmel, M., Gerdtham, U.G., Nilsson, P.M., & Saha, S. (2017). Economic burden of obesity: A systematic literature review. *International Journal of Environmental Research and Public Health, 14(4),* 435.

40. Kim, D., & Basu, A. (2016). Estimating the medical care costs of obesity in the United States: Systematic review, meta-analysis, and empirical analysis. *Value in Health (19)5,* 602-613.

41. Choi, H., Lee, J., Jang, J. (2018). Lactic acid bacteria in kimchi. In K. Park, D. Kwon, K. Lee, and S. Park (Eds.). *Korean Functional Foods: Composition, Processing, and Health Benefits.* pgs. 92-93. Boca Raton: CRC Press.

42. Kim, E.K., An, S.Y., Lee, M.S., Kim, T.H., Lee, H.K., Hwang, W.S., Choe, S.J., Kim, T.Y., Han, S.J., Kim, H.J., Kim, D.J., & Lee, K.W. (2011). Fermented kimchi reduces body weight and improves metabolic parameters in overweight and obese patients. *Nutritional Research, 31(6),* 436-43.

43. Park, K. and Ju, J. (2018). Kimchi and its health benefits. In K. Park, D. Kwon, K. Lee, and S. Park (Eds.). *Korean Functional Foods: Composition, Processing, and Health Benefits.* 43-77. Boca Raton: CRC Press.

44. Kyungsun, H., Shambhunath, B., Jing–hua, W., Bong–Soo, K., Mi, J., Kim, Eun–Jung, K. & Hojun, K. (2015). Contrasting effects of fresh and fermented kimchi consumption on gut microbiota composition and gene expression related to metabolic syndrome in obese Korean women. *Molecular Nutrition and Food Research 59(5)* 1004-1008.

45. Daniells, S. (2015, March 29). Can fermented kimchi alter the gut microbiota and influence metabolism? *NutraIngredients USA.*

46. Han, K., Bose, S., Wang, J., Kim, B. , Kim, M. J., Kim, E. and Kim, H. (2015), Contrasting effects of fresh and fermented kimchi consumption on gut microbiota composition and gene expression related to metabolic syndrome in obese Korean women. *Molecular Nutrition & Food Research, 59,* 1004-1008.

47. Islam, M.S. & Choi, H. (2009). Antidiabetic effect of Korean traditional baechu (Chinese cabbage) kimchi in a type 2 diabetes model of rats. *Journal of Medicinal Food, 12(2):* 292-297.

48. Islam, M.S. & Choi, H. (2009). Antidiabetic effect of Korean traditional baechu (Chinese cabbage) kimchi in a type 2 diabetes model of rats. *Journal of Medicinal Food, 12(2),* 292-297.

49. An, S.Y., Lee, M.S., Jeon, J.Y., Ha, E.S., Kim, T.H., Yoon, J.Y., Ok, C.O., Lee, H.K., Hwang, W.S., Choe, S.J., Han, S.J., Kim, H.J., Kim, D.J., & Lee, K.W. (2013). Beneficial effects of fresh and fermented kimchi in prediabetic individuals. *Annals of Nutrition & Metabolism 63(1-2),* 111-9.

50. Park, M.Y., Kim, J., Kim, S., & Whang, K.Y. (2018). Lactobacillus curvatus KFP419 and Leuconostoc mesenteroides subsp. mesenteroides KDK411 Isolated from kimchi ameliorate hypercholesterolemia in rats. *Journal of Medicinal Food, 21(7),* 647-653.

51. Noh, J.S., Kim, H.J., Kwon, M.J., & Song, Y.O. (2009). Active principle of kimchi, 3-(4'-hydroxyl-3',5'-dimethoxyphenyl) propionic acid, retards fatty streak formation at aortic sinus of apolipoprotein E knockout mice. *Journal of Medicinal Food, 12(6),* 1206-12.

52. Jo, S.Y., Choi, E.A., Lee, J.J., & Chang, H.C. (2015). Characterization of starter kimchi fermented with Leuconostoc kimchii GJ2 and its cholesterol-lowering effects in rats fed a high-fat and high-cholesterol diet. *Journal of the Science of Food and Agriculture, 95(13),* 2750-6.

53. Kim, H.J., Noh, J.S., & Song, Y.O. (2018). Beneficial effects of kimchi, a korean fermented vegetable food, on pathophysiological factors related to atherosclerosis. *Journal of Medicinal Food, 21(2),* 127-135.

54. Brody, D., Pratt L., & Hughes, J. (2018 February). Prevalence of depression among adults aged 20 and over: United States, 2013–2016. *Center for Disease Control and Prevention.*

55. Harvard Medical School (n.d.). The gut-brain connection. *Healthbeat.*

56. Hopkins Medicine (n.d.). The brain-gut connection. *Healthy Aging.*

57. Dinan, T., Stanton, C., Cryan, J. (2013) Psychobiotics: A novel class of psychotropic. *Biological Psychiatry 74(10),* 720–726.

58. Cho, Y., Chang, J., Chang, H. (2007) Production of gamma-aminobutyric acid (GABA) by Lactobacillus buchneri isolated from kimchi and its neuroprotective effect on neuronal cells. *Journal of Microbiology and Biotechnology. 17(1):* 104-109.

59. Cho, Y.R., Chang, J.Y., & Chang, H.C. (2007). Production of gamma-aminobutyric acid (GABA) by Lactobacillus buchneri isolated from kimchi and its neuroprotective effect on neuronal cells. *Journal of Microbiology and Biotechnology, 17(1),* 104-9.

60. Parka, S. & Baeb, J. (2016) Fermented food intake is associated with a reduced likelihood of atopic dermatitis in an adult population (Korean National Health and Nutrition Examination Survey 2012-2013). *Nutrition Research (36)2,* 125-133.

61. Ryu, B.M. (2000). Effect of kimchi on inhibition of skin aging of hairless mouse. Phd diss., Pusan National University, Busan, Korea.

62. Kim, H.J., Ju, S.Y., & Park, Y.K. (2017). Kimchi intake and atopic dermatitis in Korean aged 19-49 years: The Korea National Health and Nutrition Examination Survey 2010-2012. *Asian Pacific Journal of Clinical Nutrition, 26(5),* 914-922.

63. Kwon, M.S., Lim, S.K., Jang, J.Y., Lee, J., Park, H.K., Kim, N., Yun, M., Shin, M.Y., Jo, H.E., Oh, Y.J., Roh, S.W., & Choi, H.J. (2018). Lactobacillus sakei WIKIM30 ameliorates atopic dermatitis-like skin lesions by inducing regulatory t cells and altering gut microbiota structure in mice. *Frontiers in Immunology 9.*

64. Seung, B.P., Myung, I., Young, L., Jeung Hoon, L., Jeongheui, L., Yong-Ha, P. & Young Joon, S. (2014). Effect of emollients containing vegetable-derived lactobacillus in the treatment of atopic dermatitis symptoms: Split-body clinical trial. *Annals of Dermatology, 26(2),* 150-5.

65. Park, K. & Ju, J. (2018). Kimchi and its health benefits. In K. Park, D. Kwon, K. Lee, and S. Park (Eds.). *Korean Functional Foods: Composition, Processing, and Health Benefits* (p. 57). Boca Raton: CRC Press.

66. Song, G.H., Park, E.S., Lee, S.M., Park, D.B., & Park, K.Y. (2018). Beneficial outcomes of kimchi prepared with amtak baechu cabbage and salting in brine solution: Anticancer effects in pancreatic and hepatic cancer cells. *Journal of Environmental Pathology, Toxicology, and Oncology, 37(2),*151-161.

67. Park, K.Y., Cho, E.J., Rhee, S.H., Jung, K.O., Yi, S.J., & Jhun, B.H. (2003). Kimchi and an active component, beta-sitosterol, reduce oncogenic H-Ras(v12)-induced DNA synthesis. *Journal of Medicinal Food, 6(3),* 151-6.

68. Song, J., Lee, H. (2014) Consumption of kimchi, a salt fermented vegetable, is not associated with hypertension prevalence. *Journal of Ethnic Foods (1)1*, 8-12.

Chapter 4: How to Make Kimchi: An Overview

1. Cell Press (2015 March 3). High-salt diet could protect against invading microbes. *Science Daily*.

2. Janssens, P.L., Hursel, R., Martens, E.A., & Westerterp-Plantenga, M.S. (2013). Acute effects of capsaicin on energy expenditure and fat oxidation in negative energy balance. *PloS One, 8(7)*.

3. Rosa, A., Deiana, M., Casu, V., Paccagnini, S., Appendino, G., Ballero, M., & Dessí, M.A. (2003). Antioxidant activity of capsinoids. *Journal of Agricultural and Food Chemistry, 50(25)*, 7396-401.

4. Kang, B.K., Cho, M.S., & Park, D.S. (2016). Red pepper powder is a crucial factor that influences the ontogeny of Weissella cibaria during kimchi fermentation. *Scientific Reports 6*.

5. Jeong, S.H., Lee, H.J., Jung, J.Y., Lee, S.H., Seo, H.Y., Park, W.S., & Jeon, C.O. (2013). Effects of red pepper powder on microbial communities and metabolites during kimchi fermentation. *International Journal of Food Microbiology, 160(3)*, 252-9.

6. Amagase, H., Petesch, B.L., Matsuura, H., Kasuga, S. & Itakura, Y. (2001). Intake of garlic and its bioactive components. *The Journal of Nutrition, 31(3s)*, 955S-62S.

7. Silagy, C. & Neil, A. (1994). Garlic as a lipid lowering agent-a meta-analysis. *Journal of the Royal College of the Physicians of London, 28(1)*:39-45.

8. Arzanlou, M. (2016). Inhibition of streptococcal pyrogenic exotoxin B using allicin from garlic. *Microbial Pathogenesis, 93*, 166-71.

9. Josling, P. (2001). Preventing the common cold with a garlic supplement: a double-blind, placebo-controlled survey. *Advances in Therapy, 18(4)*, 189-93.

10. Semwal, R.B., Semwal, D.K., Combrinck, S. & Viljoen, A.M. (2015). Gingerols and shogaols: Important nutraceutical principles from ginger. *Phytochemistry 117*, 554-568.

11. Jung, J.Y., Lee, S.H., Kim, J.M., Park, M.S., Bae, J.W., Hahn, Y., Madsen, E.L., & Jeon, C.O. (2011). Metagenomic analysis of kimchi, a traditional Korean fermented food. *Applied and Environmental Microbiology, 77(7)*, 2264-74.

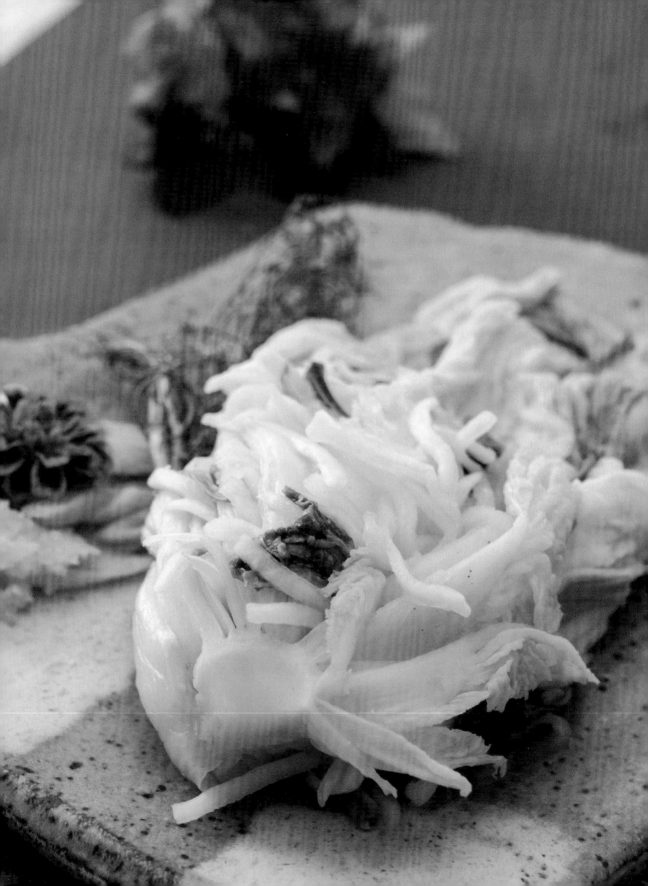

Index

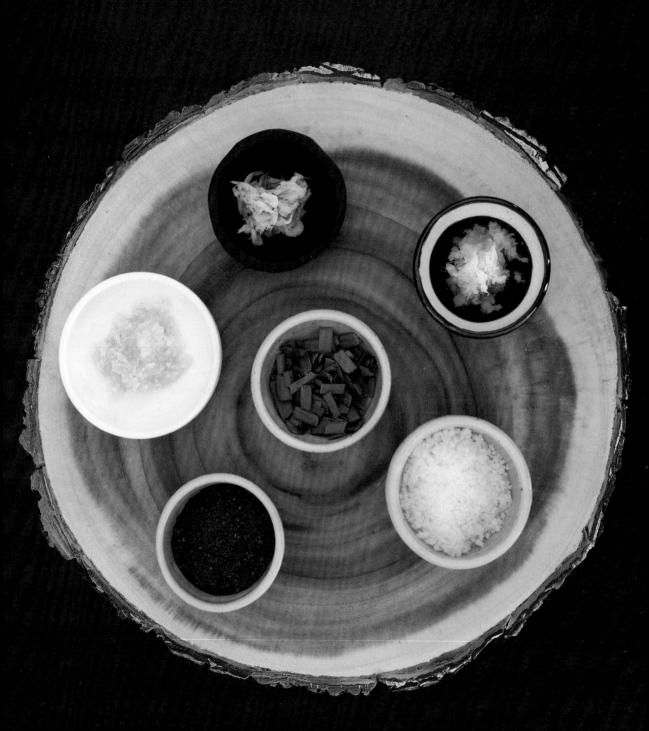

About the Author

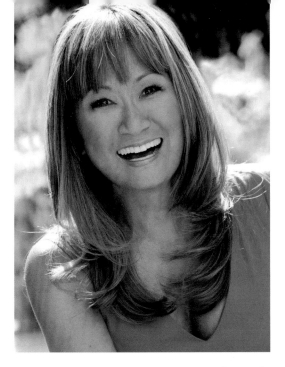

Dr. Susanne Bennett is a holistic chiropractic physician with over 30 years of clinical experience and advanced study, specializing in allergies, gut and autoimmune disorders, environmental and longevity medicine.

She's the #1 Best selling author of *Mighty Mito: Power Up Your Mitochondria for Boundless Energy, Laser Sharp Mental Focus and a Powerful Vibrant Body* and *The 7-Day Allergy Makeover: A Simple Program to Eliminate Allergies and Restore Vibrant Health from the Inside Out*.

Sharing simple health strategies to help you start feeling better today is one of Dr. Susanne's passions, and she's the dedicated talk show host of Wellness For Life on RadioMD and iHeartRadio.

As a mentor and lecturer, Dr. Susanne frequently speaks to professional and consumer audiences globally on health strategies and women's leadership.

Dr. Susanne lives in Pacific Palisades with her husband George and her pup Lola and loves organic living, snorkeling with whale sharks and eating kimchi!

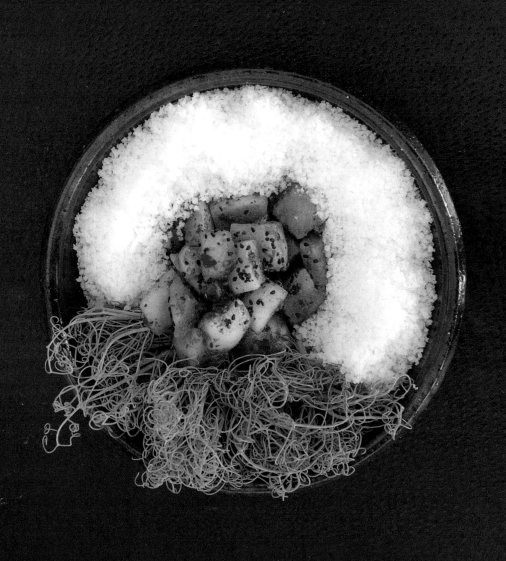